PRIMARY
FOR THE OBSTETRICIAN
AND GYNECOLOGIST

MW01168869

PRIMARY CARE FOR THE OBSTETRICIAN AND GYNECOLOGIST

Thomas E. Nolan, MD, FACOG, FACP

Associate Professor of Obstetrics and Gynecology
and Internal Medicine

Chief, Sections of General Obstetrics and Gynecology
and Critical Care Obstetrics

Louisiana State University Medical Center
New Orleans, Louisiana

WILEY-LISS

A JOHN WILEY & SONS, INC., PUBLICATION
New York • Chichester • Brisbane • Toronto • Singapore

Library of Congress Cataloging in Publication Data:

Nolan, Thomas E.
    Primary care for the obstetrician and gynecologist / Thomas E.
Nolan.
        p.   cm.
    Includes index.
    ISBN 0-471-12279-3 (alk. paper)
    1. Primary care (Medicine)   2. Women—Diseases.   3. Obstetrics.
4. Gynecology.   I. Title.
    [DNLM: 1. Primary Health Care.   2. Women's Health.   W 84 .6 N787p
1996]
RC48.6.N65   1996
616'.0082—dc20
DNLM/DLC
for Library of Congress   95-46498

Printed in the United States of America

10 9 8 7 6 5 4 3 2 1

To
Capt. Marco Labudovich, MC, USN (deceased)
Your leadership, scholarship, and unwavering dedication
to women's health care influenced a generation
of young physicians at Portsmouth Naval Hospital.
Your untimely death never allowed you to savor
the fruits of your labor.
Thanks from all your students.

► Contents

► Preface

Primary care is not a specific type of care—it is an approach to the patient and her needs, both in wellness and disease.

The goal of primary care is to treat the total patient, to maintain her health, to counsel her about risks, to prevent disease when possible, and, when disease occurs, to detect it in early stages and ensure that the care needed is provided. To be a good primary care physician is to be a good physician in the most traditional sense.

Because of changes in today's health care environment, the issue of who provides primary care has become germane. Increasingly, expensive technology has become burdensome for many patients who, perhaps naively, wish to receive more primary and preventive care. Insurance companies and third-party reimbursers are concerned that rising costs are caused by increased use of technology and diagnostic testing, although this observation has not been adequately studied or verified. As a measure of controlling costs, large health care corporations have instituted systems requiring all care to be channeled through primary care physicians. As an outgrowth of these initiatives and concerns, more physicians have been enticed to enter primary care fields—and to claim rights to the newly esteemed primary care designation.

During the health care battles of 1993 and 1994, the

American College of Obstetricians and Gynecologist became concerned that primary care issues had not been adequately addressed both in residency and in continuing medical education within the specialty. As a result, the components of primary and preventive care were identified as means of guiding further educational efforts. Even though obstetricians and gynecologist do an excellent job of caring for patients between 15 and 44 years of age, many areas have been overlooked. These deficiencies fall into areas of basic medical skills as well as in providing care for common medical conditions that are outside reproductive biology. Obstetrician–gynecologists are in a unique position to provide a full spectrum of care to patients because of the traditional focus of the specialty on routine and preventive care and the trust they have engendered in their patients on an ongoing basis. The obstetrician–gynecologist needs to become a "gate keeper" to eliminate "lock out" in the care of women. To realize this goal, an expansion of ongoing education is necessary in residency and in the "reeducation" of the practicing physician. In many areas of the country, these issues are being actively addressed and implemented.

The goal of this book is not to replace a general internal medicine textbook. It is merely meant to be a framework and quick reference for evaluation and therapies of some of the more frequent primary care problems that occur in office practice. It is not the intent of this textbook to be global, but rather to focus on key areas that can guide physicians in early detection and management of prevalent conditions that have an impact on women's health. This approach is also reflected in algorithms, which are used liberally to show a step-by-step plan for diagnosis and management. All dosages of medications are presented as currently available. However, medicine changes very quickly and readers are encouraged to confirm dosages as well as to keep abreast of emerging issues.

It is my express commitment to women's health care in obstetrics and gynecology that we offer the type of care that is both sensitive and caring as well as preventive. It is hoped that this textbook will reflect these goals and allow the obstetrician–gynecologist to continue to be the primary advocate for women.

I would like to thank Louise C. Page, editor from Wiley, for hounding (and encouraging) me to tackle this impossible project; CDR Richard Hawkins, MC, USN, a loyal internal medicine colleague who helped me through residency and agreed to proof the manuscript of this book for accuracy; and Rebecca Rinehart, whose contribution to the education of obstetricians and gynecologists through her editing has probably been underappreciated by the rank and file of ACOG.

THOMAS E. NOLAN

New Orleans, Louisiana

THE BASICS
OF PRIMARY CARE

The first two chapters establish the groundwork for primary care and the foundation on which it rests—the principles of primary and preventive care and screening. Chapter 1 is devoted to the evolution of primary care, describing economic and scientific factors that contributed to today's health care environment and why primary care has become an issue. Chapter 2 is a difficult and, in many practitioner's opinion, boring aspect of medicine: the principles of screening tests. An attempt has been made to present the concepts using real-life examples instead of mathematical models. As health networks expand and analyses of emerging information become available, screening issues will be determined not by specialty societies but by outcome data. Therefore, these issues may drive medicine, especially preventive and public health efforts, for the next decade.

The Evolution of Primary Care

Western minds are trained to "do something"—to intervene rather than to reflect. "The chance to cut is the chance to cure." This mentality is common in most physicians' psyches, especially when a specialty becomes procedure driven. The laudable goal of medicine is to eliminate disease and suffering and, paradoxically, to eliminate itself. The hardest lesson for most physicians, which some never learn, is how and when to use technology and testing. This becomes obvious in comparisons of young physicians with their older colleagues when faced with a dying patient. The philosophy of "doing everything I could" takes the physician off the emotional hook and has been a driving force in medicine in the United States. Unfortunately, when closely scrutinized, many therapies and interventions help physicians to absolve themselves of guilt rather than help patients. The interventional nature of modern medicine has supplanted preventive health care, which although often applauded is usually poorly funded. Additionally, to see the results of preventive health care in a population constantly on the move and requiring decades of study is neither satisfying nor tangible for either the physician or the patient.

For many years, health care was driven by physician's fees, which were, in most cases, arbitrarily determined. The degree of training, technical difficulty of procedures, popularity of a practice, and what the market would bear (or what insurers would reimburse) were important variables in determining compensation. The three A's of private practice—amiability, availability, and ability, in that order—continued to be major driving forces. There were no standards for outcome assessment: the surgeon who operated on low-risk patients, performing low-risk procedures, would be assumed to be a "better" surgeon in superficial comparisons. Cost control was more an issue of overhead than the type of care offered. Obstetricians and gynecologists were able to effectively market their services as the experts in the field of women's reproductive health with little resistance from other specialties. Market forces of supply and demand were of less importance than perceived "quality" of care. Many of these issues have been important for decades, especially considering that the cost of health care as a function of gross domestic product was less than 10% and not perceived as a national problem.

The 1980s were marked by an explosion of technology in testing, imaging, and surgical procedures and a corresponding explosion of profits. The cost of this care became exorbitant and, rather than consolidating technology, each center competed (and with antitrust laws in force, was forced into competition) to be the first hospital to offer services. The academic medical centers, driven by researchers whose promotion and tenure were tied to harnessing these technologies, trained more individuals to perform procedures and therapies. The extraordinary heart–lung transplant became mundane, performed in multiple medical centers at prohibitive costs. Who can deny any citizen the right to these procedures? Americans desire top-of-the-line care for every individual, regardless of their ability to pay, and at low prices. Hence the entitlement mentality of the consumer has fueled this explosion.

Despite the desire "that everything be done," little information on standardization of outcomes is available for analysis to determine who would benefit from a proposed test or procedure. The physician, buffeted by the wants and needs of the patient and trained to be an advocate regardless of ability to pay, was made responsible for cost containment. Needless to say, physicians are poorly trained to manage their own finances, let alone health care costs. Insurance companies became more interested in care provided for specific indications. This involvement has led to the creation of a bureaucracy that in most analyses has added to cost rather than contained it. The additional burden of an atmosphere heavy with litigation, in which every decision is scrutinized by attorneys whose goal is recovery and not scientific validity, has added to the need for "objective evidence" (read tests and procedures). Where is the physician to turn?

Despite the gloom and doom atmosphere prevalent in medicine today, some rays of hope are present. Money spent for elaborate technology will be consolidated within large corporations, which are buying both hospitals as well as health care provider resources. The science of testing and screening will no longer be in the domain of the academic medical center, influenced by the inherent bias of the populations served, but will be generated by outcome analysis. This methodology removes the physician from offering certain services. The modern obstetrician–gynecologist will have to learn how to effectively gather data on outcomes and prove that care rendered is appropriate and beneficial. In many ways, this approach could allow the physician to become free of some technology that has been advocated by national organizations and to focus on issues germane to patient care.

Technology may be helpful in delivering health care in new and unique ways. Medical recordkeeping and retrieval are archaic at best. Every new patient seeking care from a provider comes with little information relating to prior services rendered, ongoing problems, medications, and family history. Added to the confusion is the manner in which the information is presented to the provider. One needs only to request narrative summaries and operative reports to reveal how little many very intelligent patients understood of the care they received. Valuable time is wasted collecting redundant data rather than "connecting" with the patient on such relevant issues as work, family, and the inherent stresses of life. If properly designed, the use of standardized forms and computer databases will allow a patient and her physician quick access to medical records. They may also signal when an immunization is indicated and when preventive testing should be initiated.

What do all these issues have to do with primary care? Patients (not clients!) prefer to have a single provider with whom they work well and feel comfortable. Traditionally, obstetrician–gynecologists have been women's health care advocates and most women would prefer receiving care from physicians in the specialty. Unfortunately, as medical education has changed, so too has the specialty, which in many ways has narrowed. Economic and political forces are *demanding* primary care physicians become decision makers and, consequently, are steering patients toward the cheapest and most effective provider. For obstetrics and gynecology to survive as a specialty in the current scope of care, it must change from a procedure-based specialty and become more focused on total patient care. Total patient care requires that physicians, who may be uncomfortable caring for some common diseases, expand the care they offer. Once the patient leaves the practice, the provider may never see that patient again. Unfortunately, other specialties have not been active in women's health care. For obstetricians and gynecologists to continue to remain competitive, we will need to return to basic "doctoring" skills and the care of common diseases. We are capable of assuming this role and have a tradition of doing so. This book provides the preparation for a basic approach to primary care and it is hoped will help relieve some of the anxiety associated with change.

CHAPTER 2

Principles of Screening

Screening is the assessment of the risk of a disorder occurring in individuals or a population with no evidence of disease. Screening operates at various levels and requires that for each patient a reliable history is obtained and physical examination is performed during the initial visit. This allows the practitioner to selectively utilize available resources and testing for individual patients rather than using an "all or nothing" approach. It also enables the practitioner to obtain critical information prior to ordering a test or therapy. In the near future, it is hoped that patient data will be handled electronically, allowing the practitioner to assess aspects of the history that are germane, medications and surgical procedures the patient has received, and immunizations that are needed.

Screening can identify patients who are at high or low risk of a disease, allowing further testing to be focused based on risk factors. It allows disease to be detected in early stages and promotes preventive care and early intervention. Principles of screening, outlined in this chapter, are applicable within the broad range of primary and preventive care.

► BENEFITS AND LIMITATIONS

Screening can encompass a history, physical examination, and laboratory tests. Generally, however, it is considered testing individuals who have no evidence of disease. It can also apply to testing in individuals who do not have signs and symptoms of a disease but who are identified as being at high risk for a disorder based on certain characteristics.

Screening can identify individuals who are free of disease or at low risk for the development of a disease. The value of some tests is to provide reassurance to patients. A good example of such use is normal mammography results in a woman with a strong family history of breast cancer whose breast self-examination and clinical examination results are normal.

Screening can identify individuals who are susceptible to the development of a disease. Health care workers who have a questionable history of childhood varicella exposure and who lack the antibody may receive a vaccine when entering the workplace. The Pap test may be performed more often in patients who are at increased risk of cervical carcinoma such as immunocompromised individuals taking medication for transplantation or connective tissue disorders or those with human immunodeficiency virus (HIV) infection.

Screening can identify a patient with a precursor of a disease. Individuals with cancer of the reproductive tract are more susceptible to other cancers, such as breast cancer. Additionally, individuals who were cured of one malignancy with radiation or chemotherapy are at higher risk of associated carcinomas, such as thyroid cancer following neck irradiation for Hodgkin's disease or leukemia following chemotherapy.

Screening can identify individuals with a disease or condition before it becomes clinically manifest. In certain diseases, such as colorectal carcinoma, malignant melanoma, and breast cancer, the chance of survival has a direct relationship to the stage in which therapy is initiated. Therefore, use of screening fecal occult blood testing and screening mammography to detect nonpalpable breast cancer will detect the disease before metastases have occurred.

Screening may identify individuals who have a disease or who pose a risk to others. The screening and surveillance of sexually transmitted diseases and treatment of consorts are based on epidemiologic principles. Recently, it has been shown that the treatment of HIV-infected mothers with zidovudine can lower the risk of fetal and neonatal infection. Identification of maternal hepatitis infection may stop the vertical transmission of infection to the fetus as well as allow prophylaxis and treatment of family members in close contact.

The benefit of screening is based on the prevalence of the disorder and the sensitivity of tests. Therefore, the value of screening must be assessed within the limits of the accuracy of the screening tests, which have confidence limits and are stratified, as are populations under study.

▶ TESTING

Tests for screening should be evaluated for their usefulness and limitations in terms of accuracy, risks, and cost. The physician should use such information to assess what can be expected from the test. A mathematical determination can be used to define these issues in the following terms:

Sensitivity. The ability of a test or procedure to identify individuals *with* the disease.

Specificity. The ability of a test or procedure to identify persons *without* the disease.

Positive Predictive Value. The likelihood that a positive test result will identify persons *with* the disease.

Negative Predictive Value. The likelihood that a negative test result will identify persons *without* the disease.

What does this mean to the harried practitioner? Sensitivity and specificity are important to the epidemiologist or public health official in determining what test will have the greatest value when used on a screening basis. Also, it explains why some tests are "good" tests for screening or why some individuals will have serologic evidence of disease without actually having the disease. Predictive values are of importance to the clinician who is taking care of individuals on a smaller scale and must make therapeutic decisions based on test results. Predictive values are driven by the population (i.e., patients), whereas sensitivity and specificity are driven by the accuracy of the test.

Test results should be assessed within the context of predictive values; otherwise, results can be misinterpreted. An example of misinterpreting the value of a laboratory test is the problem with Lyme's disease in the southern United States. Lyme's disease was first described and named after the area of Connecticut in which it was first discovered. Because of the proximity of this area to major teaching institutions, the endemic was described with a tick vector, and laboratory tests were developed. The rate of false-positive results of the test was 0.1%, which means the that if 1000 individuals without the disease had the laboratory test, one person would have positive test results without having the disease. Lyme's disease was found to be a cause of chronic arthritis. The stigma of chronic diseases, especially those without a well-known cause, raises the spectrum of malingering and frustrates patients and physicians. When Lyme's disease became publicized, patients demanded to know if they had this malady. In the deep South, where the vector of disease is rare, the incidence was in the range of 0.01% to 0.001% (1:10,000 to 1:100,000). If all the individuals with suspected disease were tested, the incidence of laboratory disease (i.e., a false-positive result) is greater than the actual incidence of the disease. However, if the individual had a history of the characteristic rash, the possibility of actual disease being present increases dramatically. Therefore, the clinician should be responsible for understanding screening issues and test appropriately, rather than testing whole populations with a low incidence of the disease.

The value of a test used in a population is affected by how many persons in that population have the disease. The recent controversy in such ares as frequency of Pap testing and initiation mammography testing are prime examples of the dilemma facing the clinician in evaluating testing schemes.

Cost effectiveness is an important aspect of the value of screening. Unfortunately, it is often politicized based on ethical or philosophic considerations. The Agency for Health Care Policy and Research is a federal agency that is attempting to assemble evidence related to these issues. However, each issue studied costs $1.2 million and has limited widespread utilization. All screening tests should be subjected to thorough review to allow valid conclusions to be reached and tests to be performed without outside influence. In the absence of such high-quality (but expensive) information, decisions will continue to be made on the basis of best judgment. Therefore, health care providers and the public must expect some disagreement in the various documents that currently address various screening techniques.

The disagreement between the American Cancer Society and the American College of Obstetricians and Gynecologists is a prime example of the controversy regarding the frequency of routine Pap tests. In terms of dollars spent in screening, following are the basic issues to be addressed:

- *What does it cost to identify one case correctly in comparison to the cost to those persons incorrectly identified by the test?* A significant number of individuals have low-titer antibodies in laboratory determinations for systemic lupus erythematosus (SLE). Although these individuals do not have the disease, they are labeled as having it. Many of the laboratory tests are made from different cell lines (all tests are not created equal!) and have varying thresholds for what constitutes normal and abnormal results. Finally, some individuals with positive test results will progress to clinical disease, whereas some do not. The underlying principle is: SLE is uncommon and the number of false-positive results in screening limits the value of certain laboratory studies.

- *Is there a benefit to a person who was correctly identified?* An 80-year-old patient with end-stage ovarian disease will derive no benefit from a work-up for a positive fecal occult blood test.

- *Is there a risk to a person incorrectly identified (invasive testing)?* An individual with a false-positive fecal occult blood test result may undergo colonoscopy, resulting in the perforation of an existing diverticulum because the examiner did not recognize it: the patient undergoes a double-barrel colostomy and reanastomosis 8 weeks later.

• *What does testing mean when applied to a large population?* A known risk factor for cervical carcinoma is male–female penile vaginal intercourse with multiple partners. Are there benefits to annual Pap testing for monogamous lesbians?

Criteria for evaluating a test, especially if it is used for large screening programs, should be assessed. Is there one test (not necessarily the screening test) that is the "gold standard"? The Western blot is the gold standard in HIV diagnosis, but it is time consuming and expensive. Therefore, the ELISA (enzyme-linked immunoadsorbent assay) test is used for screening (cheap with very good sensitivity and specificity), with results confirmed by Western blot. This is also called "sequencing," where screening moves to a confirmatory test. Test results should also be reproducible and have a "normal" level that is defined. The setting of the test should be stated, such as how measurement of blood pressure is performed. Finally, are the tactics that are used in a testing scheme defined in a clear fashion, and does utility of the test allow the individual to benefit from the results?

Many of the advances in screening will be in the use of tests in individuals or populations who do not have manifestations of the disease but are identified as being at high risk for the disorder because of a distinctive characteristic. In the current health care environment, testing may be mandated by large corporations such as health maintenance organizations. These organizations, if data acquisition and management are properly applied, may help in structuring testing schemes. For instance, as familial and genetic characteristics of colorectal carcinoma are better identified, chromosomal testing may help identify high-risk individuals, eliminating testing in low-risk individuals. Currently, the presence of a high-risk factor may be the primary indication for screening. In the future, screening may be stratified by characteristics that influence, for example, the age at which screening is started or the frequency of testing. Identification of high-risk factors by means of an expanded history and physical examination is not limited to medical issues. Social, occupational and behavioral aspects of the history are becoming of increasing importance in assessing overall risks and general health.

▶ PERIODIC ASSESSMENTS

Subsequent periodic evaluations are a part of continuing care. In Chapter 5, a modified version of the United States Preventative Services Task Force recommendations for routine screening and assessment is presented. These recommendations represent initial attempts to address issues in screening and will undergo substantial modification over the next several years. As the results of outcome studies emerge, screening will become a dynamic force in medical care as defined by goals of prevention of disease. Periodic evaluations are planned as scheduled appointments for asymptomatic patients and may be incorporated easily into the annual pelvic examination. Currently, the specific schedule is based on a patient's needs and the physician's discretion, but in the future it may be determined by health maintenance organizations.

WELLNESS, HEALTH PROMOTION, AND HEALTH MAINTENANCE

As mortality rates from infectious diseases have decreased, the average age of the population has increased. With this change in demographics, disease patterns have changed. Cancer and chronic diseases have become more important in overall morbidity and mortality. The ability to make an impact on many diseases, such as cancer and diabetes, is directly related to either the stage of disease at discovery or control of environmental factors such as diet. To detect diseases at an earlier stage, when interventions may save lives or modify disease course, screening has assumed greater importance.

Chapter 3 deals with important aspects of wellness such as immunizations, nutrition, and exercise. Physicians born and educated prior to the availability of many modern immunizations remember vividly the effect these infections had on populations. As a single health issue, immunizations have had a major impact. Newer agents, such as hepatitis B and varicella vaccines, will continue to improve the health and well-being of society in general. Nutrition is probably one the most important health issues in the United States and probably the least understood by many physicians. Additionally, many individuals are preparing less food at home and consequently eating more fast food. Issues such as fats in the diet are being linked causally to cancers such as breast and colon. Effective counseling on diet and exercise or the recognition of dietary problems and referral to a dietitian may alter many chronic diseases, especially diabetes, hypertension, hypercholesterolenemia, cardiovascular risk, and osteoarthritis. Therefore, nutritional issues are becoming more important to general health and wellness. Finally, the positive effects of exercise and its benefit in preventing such diverse conditions as coronary artery disease and constipation are being recognized.

Chapter 4 focuses on office counseling. At the height of sexual awareness in the late 1960s and early 1970s, counseling was very popular. However, the increase in sexually transmitted diseases and human immunodeficiency virus, as well as questions about the propriety of many "sexual" counselors, has reduced the number of qualified individuals. Obstetrician–gynecologists will need to fill the void with regard to counseling about sexuality as well as other psychosocial factors that contribute to general health. They will also need to expand their role in other areas such as accident prevention, domestic violence, and substance abuse, all of which have a significant impact on morbidity and mortality. This chapter will present a paradigm to assist in modifying behavior.

Chapter 5 is a compendium of previously released material on preventive health care and current screening strategies promoted by the United States Public Health Task Force. Many of the issues discussed in Section 1, specifically screening, will change as outcome data become available. Many of the recommendations were made by governing organizations whose primary focus is certain diseases and their treatment. In the next 5 years, many of the recommendations will probably be modified.

CHAPTER 3

Preventive Medicine

Disease prevention and the concept of wellness have become more important than treatment. The concept of wellness is a basic approach to life that encompasses diet, weight control, and exercise. Other aspects include avoidance of premature deaths by accident prevention and disease prevention by immunization and life-style adjustments such as smoking cessation and moderation in alcohol consumption. Weight control alone can help prevent such diseases as diabetes[1] and hence heart disease. Dietary control of fats also can help reduce weight and, in susceptible individuals, heart disease. Exercise may help promote better bowel function and prevent heart disease through high-density lipoprotein enhancement. Finally, periodic screening for silent diseases such as hypertension will help eliminate premature atherosclerosis and renal disease. The practitioner's primary scope may change from disease recognition to prevention, which will require a change in perception by both the patient and provider.

▶ IMMUNIZATIONS

Immunizations consist of three major classes: vaccines, toxoids, and immunoglobulins, which are defined as follows[2]:

1. *Vaccines.* A suspension of attenuated live or killed microorganisms (bacteria, viruses, or rickettsiae), or fractions thereof, administered to induce immunity and prevent infections.

2. *Toxoid.* A modified bacterial toxin that has been rendered nontoxic but retains the ability to stimulate the formation of antitoxin.

3. *Immunoglobin.* Subdivided into general and specific:
   a) *Generalized.* A sterile solution for intramuscular administration containing antibody from human blood. It is primarily indicated for routine protection of certain immunodeficient persons and for passive immunization against measles and hepatitis A. Additionally, intravenous administration of immunoglobin is indicated for replacement therapy in IgG deficiency and idiopathic thrombocytopenic purpura.
   b) *Specific.* Special preparations obtained from pools of serum with known high quantities of antibody for specific infections. These include hepatitis B immune globulin (HBIG) for hepatitis B infection, varicella zoster immune globulin (VZIG) for varicella infections, rabies immune globulin (RIG) for rabies infection, and tetanus immune globulin (TIG) for tetanus infections.

   Guidelines for therapy are as follows:

All Groups

- *Tetanus–Diphtheria Booster.* Should be administered every 10 years.

- *Influenza Vaccine.* Annually beginning at age 55 and for high-risk groups including health care workers and individuals with chronic cardiovascular and pulmonary diseases (including asthma). Other candidates include persons with renal insufficiency, diabetes mellitus, and immunosuppression.

- *Pneumococcal Vaccine.* A one-time vaccine that contains 23 of 28 possible serotypes. It should be given at age 65 and repeated at 6 years in high-risk individuals. High-risk groups include those with cardiopulmonary disease or asplenic individuals resulting from either trauma or autolysis from hemoglobinopathies. Currently, it is unknown if this vaccine is safe in pregnancy.[3]

High-Risk Groups

- *Mumps, Measles, Rubella.* Females of childbearing age lacking evidence of immunity should receive a rubella vaccine. If possible, this vaccine should be given prior to pregnancy in nonimmune women. A second measles immunization, preferably as MMR (measles–mumps–rubella vaccine), should be given to all women unable to show proof of immunity. Mumps vaccine should not be given during pregnancy.

- *Hepatitis B.* Vaccine should be given to all health care providers. Other high-risk individuals include intravenous drug users, current recipients of blood products, persons in health-related jobs with exposure to blood or blood products, household and sexual contacts with HBV carriers, sexually active persons with multiple sexual partners diagnosed as having recently acquired sexually transmitted diseases, prostitutes, and persons who have a history of sexual activity with multiple partners in the previous 6 months. All infants are currently vaccinated and consideration should be given to vaccination of adolescents.

- *Hepatitis A.* Vaccine has recently been approved (Spring 1995. Groups considered at high risk are health care and sanitation workers and international travelers (military) in areas with poor sanitation.

- *Varicella.* Vaccine also has recently been approved (Spring 1995). Infants will be the first group for primary mass immunization. Individuals at high risk such as health care workers without evidence of immunologic conversion will also be considered candidates. Controversy exists on how effective the vaccine will be over a lifetime (i.e., will individuals vaccinated as a child be protected after 50 or 60 years).

▶ NUTRITION AND WEIGHT CONTROL

Patients who require nutritional counseling are not necessarily motivated by weight control, but rather by an interest in improved appearance. Obesity has become a progressive health problem in the United States with 35% of nonpregnant women classified as overweight.[4] In the other extreme, younger women, many with eating disorders such as bulimia or anorexia nervosa, may be encountered. Vegetarians are usually well informed concerning nutrition but require occasional monitoring, whereas those following more extreme diets, in which eggs and milk products are restricted, may require close assessment during counseling. Certain ethnic groups are at higher risk such as Mexican–American and African–American women.

Diet has assumed greater importance in the past decade as information has emerged regarding the relationship between various foods and weight gain and their influence on cardiovascular disease, diabetes, certain cancers, and osteoporosis. In the past, most medical aspects of nutritional assessment focused on avoiding chronic deficiencies and disease states. Less important but still of concern is the amelioration of existing diseases and vitamin deficiencies. Both viewpoints are not mutually exclusive and relate to the individual perceptions of quality of life. In lower socioeconomic groups, however, relative protein deficiencies may be present as well as iron deficiency anemia. The American diet still remains higher in fats and lower in fiber than optimal recommendations. To assess nutritional needs in the outpatient environment, screening, counseling, diagnosis, and management need to be integrated so that a program can be implemented. The clinician should be aware that recommended daily allowances (RDAs) change periodically and are adjusted for age and gender.

Screening

Current dietary practices should be reviewed for dietary excesses and possible deficiencies. A common misperception is that obese patients are not malnourished and are nutritionally replete. Other aspects of nutritional counseling are reinforcing appropriate eating practices, identifying inappropriate practices requiring remedial care, correcting misinformation, and identifying disease states. These guidelines allow the physician to determine which patients need additional in-depth assessment. Additionally, risk factors for poor nutrition should be identified such as age (adolescence and the elderly, especially those living alone), low income, cigarette or substance abuse, pica and frequent dieting, skipping meals, and vegan diets. Medical conditions that contribute to poor nutrition include mental illness with psychosis or major depression, muscle weakness involving the muscle of mastication, and certain medications, such as phenytoin, which may result in vitamin deficiencies.

Opening questions can be asked about the patient's attitude toward her body image, weight, and weight distribution. A 24-hour diet recall history or a diary will provide information about food intake, meals eaten, and meals skipped. Recent weight changes should be documented as well as intake of such items as alcohol, vitamin and mineral supplements, candy, and soft drinks. Some patients should be asked if they have sufficient money to buy food and to refrigerate and prepare food. A simple questionnaire may be obtained from the hospital nutritionist or formulated to the specific characteristics of the population served.

Diagnosis

History is the most important assessment tool in the diagnosis of illness related to inadequate or inappropriate diet. A questionnaire may be administered by ancillary personnel for initial interviewing and assessment of patients. Once the responses are reviewed, the practitioner may investigate areas of particular interest. Clues derived from the patient may be reinforced by findings on physical examination. Of particular importance on physical examination are distribution of body fat and signs of malnutrition such as oral cavity diseases (poor dentition with periodontal diseases) and skin diseases.

Weight related to height will provide body mass index or BMI (kg/m^2). This calculation should be coupled with clinical judgment to conclude that large boned or muscular individuals or very petite individuals may be outside the normal ranges and thus not be obese or malnourished. Evaluation of the distribution of fat and muscle mass is the most practical way to assess normal, overweight, and underweight categories. Although obesity and anorexia may easily be recognized, the bulimic patient may have a normal body habitus. Recently, body distribution of fat has been described by using the waist/hip ratio, as summarized:

- Measure the waist with a nonstretchable tape in a horizontal plane at just above the right ilium on the midaxillary line. For practical purposes, this is the area just below the smallest area of the "waist."

- Measure the hips at the maximum posterior extension between the iliac crest and buttocks.

- Divide the waist measurement by the hip measurement. A value approaching or exceeding 1 suggests increased health risk greater than expected by excessive weight alone.[5]

Blood chemistry levels usually are not helpful in the evaluation of malnutrition. If testing is considered, most laboratories offer a series that may include albumin, transferrin, retinol-binding protein, and thyroxine-binding prealbumin. Leukopenia and the presence of both megaloblastic and microcytic anemia are indicative of advanced malnutrition. Lipid profiles should be offered to patients with a family history of cardiovascular disease. Laboratory tests should be performed to rule out endocrine disorders if there is a clinical suspicion derived from personal or family history, physical examination, or risk factors (i.e., ethnic group). These tests and indications are discussed in later chapters.

Counseling

Great diversity exists in the diets and eating habits of Americans, which are specific to cultural, ethnic, and religious backgrounds.[6] Therefore, important influences unknown to the provider may be operative and difficult to modify unless the practitioner is aware and culturally sensitive to these issues. Regardless of dietary preferences, there are tenets of healthful nutrition that are applicable to all individuals. Unfortunately, in the United States, regardless of race, education, or income, most people do not follow these guidelines. Most patients will benefit from current information about nutrition, healthful diet composition, and, in many cases, weight control. Additionally, women may have specific needs such as folic acid use preconceptionally, iron intake in menstruating women, and calcium intake in patients at high risk for osteoporosis.

Recommendations for the maintenance of good health include ingesting daily:

- Thirty percent or less of daily caloric intake as fat with less than 10% of calories as saturated fatty acid
- Five or more daily servings of fruits and vegetables
- Six or more daily servings of starches and complex carbohydrates
- Moderate levels of protein
- Less than 1 ounce of pure alcohol

- Sodium intake of 6 g or less
- Food containing adequate calcium and iron content

In the outpatient environment, the most efficient way to accomplish dietary education is by providing selected written materials. The materials should be specific to the patient's needs and background, if possible.

Individuals at high risk for malnutrition may be casualties of food faddism, low and high body mass index, and medical diseases (i.e., Crohn's disease, ulcerative colitis, malignancies). Special dietary requirements, the presence of low and high body mass index, and other states that may affect intake or absorption require intense and knowledgeable counseling to effect change. A thorough and detailed history should be obtained from the patient. Core data include an assessment of the patient's present goals, a willingness to change, previous attempts to change and motivation for change. Additionally, other aspects should be discussed such as the family's willingness to change and initiation of a exercise program. Finally, all points of contact with food should be discussed including shopping for food, methods of preparation, when the food is consumed, and the quantities eaten.

Management

Management may prove difficult unless the patient perceives there is a problem and is willing to modify all aspects of nutrition. In most instances, remedial actions involve a combination of changes in amount and type of food eaten, implementation of a fitness program, and behavior modification therapy. Success in obtaining permanent change is enhanced when mutual agreement by patient and provider is reached and the following realistic goals are established:

- A weight endpoint
- Time frame for change (e.g., 5 pounds a month)
- A commitment to long-term maintenance of dietary change and exercise program endpoints

The provider should offer positive feedback and reinforcement rather than negative feedback and assess barriers and patient constraints that need to be overcome. Frequently, referral to other health professionals (primarily dietitians) and peer support groups is necessary. Additionally, the practitioner should be willing to see the patient periodically and offer support and insight. Effective counseling techniques, especially for patients challenged with stressful situations, are important in maintaining weight control. Finally, weight control is usually a life-long battle and the supportive role of the practitioner should never be underappreciated or understated.

► EXERCISE

The effects of exercise and its contribution to a healthy lifestyle have become more evident as increasing evidence suggests that wellness requires some element of physical exertion.[7] Exercise is a major component of "fitness," a broad term that encompasses cardiovascular fitness, endurance, and weight control. Exercise has become an important aspect of daily living for many women for these reasons as well as for stress reduction. As part of an overall wellness program, questions concerning the amount of exercise the patient performs on a weekly basis should be acquired and recorded. An active exercise program should be recommended for individuals with a sedentary life.

Cardiovascular fitness occurs when the body increases its aerobic *capacity* by increasing oxygen storage capacity at the cellular level. A major by-product of the increase in aerobic capacity is the ability to prolong the capacity for physical activity ("conditioning") that results in more energy for exercises and daily activities.[8] An exercise program is an important aspect in weight loss and control and increases the effectiveness of any program. For the average patient, the main goals of an exercise program are usually a combination of cardiovascular fitness and weight control. In addition, exercise may increase muscle strength, flexibility, and coordination. Weight-bearing exercises and high-intensity strength training may also increase bone density, an important factor in preventing osteoporosis.[9]

Cardiovascular Fitness

Oxygen storage capacity increases with the duration of exercise and is referred to as "conditioning." In the laboratory, this response is called aerobic capacity and is measured by determining maximum oxygen uptake (Vo_2 max). Eventually, if exercise is continued, oxygen capabilities are exceeded and lactic acid is produced. Because both of these measures require extensive laboratory support, heart rate is substituted for its ease of measurement. Heart rate is an excellent method to evaluate cardiovascular fitness and estimate the Vo_2 max. As cardiovascular fitness improves, the heart rate will stabilize at a fixed rate of exercise determined by multiple factors, including age. It is possible to establish the heart rate at which conditioning will develop by using the following formula to determine the target range:

$$(220 - \text{age}) \times 60\text{–}80\% = \text{Target Range}$$

For example, a 55-year-old patient would have a target range of 99 to 132 ($220 - 55 = 165 \times 0.6 = 99$ or $\times 0.8 = 132$ beats per minute). To achieve physical fitness, an exercise program needs to maintain the heart rate within these parameters. To attain minimal cardiovascular fitness, a woman must exercise at a level that elevates the heart rate into her age-adjusted target range for 20 minutes or more, at least three times a week. Warm-up and cool-down periods should be used to prevent muscle injury and allow the cardiovascular system to adjust. The warm-up period, which slowly increases blood supply to peripheral large muscle groups and helps prevent muscle injury, should last approximately 5 minutes. Similarly, the cool-down period allows blood in the skin and muscles to return to the central vasculature, thus preventing dizziness, nausea, and fainting as the heart rate returns to normal.

Weight Control

Weight loss from exercise occurs if more calories are used than ingested and the resulting deficit modifies existing fat stores. Therefore, for an exercise program to be effective for weight control, a negative caloric balance must be achieved (i.e., caloric intake must be less than calories expended). Each pound of body fat contains 3500 calories. If 500 calories are expended daily and caloric intake remains stable, 1 pound a week will be lost. As fat is lost, in many cases muscle mass increases. Since muscle weighs twice as much as fat, there may be negligible weight loss in the early stages of the program. Despite this, clothing may drop in size or fit better. Meaningful weight loss takes time and this should be emphasized when the program is initiated. The patient's weight should be evaluated and recorded on a regular basis and progress in exercise and weight loss discussed.

Developing a Program

Just as a diet will be successful only if individual needs are met, so too does the success of an exercise program depend on satisfaction of needs. Goals should be predetermined and reasonable so that specific encouragement and recommendations may be offered. Patients under age 45 with no history of chronic illness or injury do not require a physical examination or special laboratory tests before beginning an exercise program. After age 45, a lipid profile and electrocardiogram are recommended as a baseline to determine any evidence of ischemia or prior myocardial infarctions. Regardless of the type of program the patient undertakes, she should be cautioned about the warning signs of overexertion:

- Irregular heart beat
- Excessive fatigue, dizziness, or faintness
- Difficulty breathing
- Nausea, vomiting
- Excessive muscle pain or any sharp pain

Should any of these signs occur, the patient should stop exercising and contact her doctor for follow-up or evaluation, especially if cardiac disease is suspected.

Activities that are commonly recommended include brisk walking, jogging, running, bicycling, cross-country skiing, stair stepping or machine exercises, swimming, and aerobics. Other sports such as racquetball, tennis, and volleyball are beneficial if they require continuous activity for 20 minutes or more without intermittent rest periods. There are now numerous opportunities in most communities to enroll in an exercise program. Aerobic classes of various levels and intensity are widely available. Low-impact aerobics are probably best suited for pregnant patients and older peri- and postmenopausal women. An increase in sport medicine injuries has been reported in middle-age individuals, so exercise programs should be designed to avoid muscle, ligament, and bone injury. Indoor exercise machines are excellent sources of physical activity in a secure, protected environment. Additionally, they allow the participant to read, listen to music, or watch television while exercising. Circuit training, which is a predefined program of exercises, is available in many city parks and recreation areas. In most cases, they combine running, climbing, pulling, pushing, and jumping. Weight training programs should be developed for those individuals who desire strength training. These programs are best developed with and supervised by trained instructors.

The program should match the needs of the patient. Many women currently work and are raising a family. If possible, programs should be designed to fit into an already hectic schedule. Follow-up should not only target the exercise and weight aspects of conditioning but also promote dietary goals as well. Finally, exercise may have some role in the prevention of osteoporosis.

► REFERENCES

1. Manson JE, Rimm EB, Stampfer MJ, et al. Physical activity and incidence of non-insulin-dependent diabetes mellitus in women. *Lancet* 1991;338:774–8.

2. Centers for Disease Control and Prevention. Recommendation of the Immunization Practices Advisory Committee (ACIP): general recommendations on immunization. *MMWR Morb Mortal Wkly Rep* 1194;43(RR-1).

3. Centers for Disease Control and Prevention. Recommendation of the Immunization Practices Advisory Committee (ACIP): pneumococcal vaccine. *MMWR Morb Mortal Wkly Rep* 1989;64–8,73–6.

4. Kuczmarski RJ, Flegal KM, Campbell SM, Johnson CL. Increasing prevalence of overweight among US adults: The National Health and Nutrition Examination Surveys, 1960–1991. *JAMA* 1994;272:205–11.

5. Chumlea WC, Kuczmarski RJ. Using a bony landmark to measure waist circumference. *J Am Diet Assoc* 1995;95:12.

6. Kant AK, Block G, Schatzkin A, Ziegler RG, Nestle M. Dietary diversity in the US population, NHANES II, 1976–1980. *J Am Diet Assoc* 1991;91:1526–1531.

7. Smith CW Jr. Exercise: a practical guide for helping the patient achieve a health lifestyle. *J Am Board Fam Pract* 1989;2:238–46.

8. *ACOG Technical Bulletin* 1992;173. Oct

9. Nelson ME, Fiatarone MA, Morganti CM, Trice I, Greenberg RA, Evans WJ. Effects of high-intensity strength training on multiple risk factors for osteoporotic fractures: a randomized controlled trial. *JAMA* 1994;272:1909–14.

Counseling

Counseling in the office environment is as much an art form as a science. The sensitivity, empathy, and insight of the examining physician are essential in eliciting an accurate history and implementing therapy. Because of the flexible nature of human interaction, multiple theories and conventions in counseling have been offered. The most common counseling therapies in sexual dysfunction include marital–family therapy, interactional therapy, behavioral therapy, and cognitive therapy.

Early Freudian and psychoanalytic therapies concentrated on developmental stages in life and continue to influence modern counseling. The major premise in the Freudian theory of sexual dysfunction was that any deviation in development led to aberrant sexual development. Additionally, resolution of Oedipal conflict was required for appropriate sexual function to occur; these concepts were operative until Master's and Johnson's breakthrough book.[1] Starting in the 1960s, the introduction of the birth control pill and the so-called sexual revolution led to multiple schools of thought.[2] Unfortunately, may self-described experts and practitioners of sexual behavior therapy began to practice, using trendy psychoanalysis. After misuse of these therapies became widespread and their effectiveness was questioned, many patients and physicians became

37

wary. Currently, there are a limited number of responsible practitioners in this field.

The behavioral schools have become more popular in the past 30 years and, considering the nature of the busy outpatient environment, are probably more practical in general counseling as well as sexual counseling. In resistant and difficult cases, referral to practitioners in the more traditional schools of psychiatry should be considered. In the initial assessment, the patient should be assured that she is not psychotic or profoundly neurotic. Additionally, the practitioner should feel comfortable with the patient and avoid transference, especially in issues of sexual dysfunction.

Theories of Change

Current counseling techniques incorporate the best of different therapeutic efforts into a new framework of thought involving the concepts or "science" of *change*.[3] The core of these teachings deals with the persistence of various behaviors and how they effect change in human affairs. Central to this thought was the failure of common sense and logic in some problem solving, while at times illogical and unreasonable approaches are successful. This observation has led to a better understanding of the role or art of the effective counselor in using different approaches to effect change. This alternate method of counseling to effect change emphasized the use of metaphors and *interventional* suggestions rather than classic passive insights.[4]

Diagnosis

Counseling should reach certain endpoints, most importantly to effect a therapeutic response. Ten steps recommended by the United States Preventative Services Task Force are the following:

1. Develop a therapeutic alliance.
2. Counsel all patients.
3. Ensure that patients understand the relationship between behavior and health.
4. Work with patients to assess barriers to behavior change.
5. Gain commitment from patients to change.
6. Involve patients in selecting risk factors.
7. Use a combination of strategies.
8. Design a behavior modification factor.
9. Monitor progress through follow-up contact.
10. Involve office staff.

Once a problem is identified that requires more extensive counseling, another appointment should be made with sufficient time for free discussion. Change therapy is behavioral therapy that stresses that contemporary events, as well as how the different individuals relate to the event, must be understood by all involved parties.[3] Most individuals who seek therapy have self-initiated an extensive effort to discover and implement a "cure" for their problem. Clarifying the self-perceived "problem" as envisioned and described by the patient is the first step in therapy.

Other steps necessary in the initial assessment include the following:

• Documenting the steps the patient has taken in resolving the problem

- Determining what efforts have helped or hindered in the process (fortunately, many self-described "solutions" to problems in fact represent part of the problem!)

- Finding and correcting medical or gynecologic problems (e.g., herpes simplex type II in vaginismus and vulvadynia)

- Broadening horizons to avoid focusing or overamplification of unrelated situations

- Debunking myths, especially important in sexual dysfunction therapy, and eliminating misinformation regarding utopias (common in weight loss schemes)

- Redirecting, often with paradoxical suggestions (you have sexual dysfunction: rather than continued effort for intercourse—stop all efforts)

- Recommending selected readings to educate the patient to assist in reframing thought processes

- Enhancing communication, particularly important in sexual and family dysfunction

All these methodologies are standard therapy methods useful in creating change. There at least two levels of change referred to as *first* and *second* order:

- First order change is characterized as superficial and mechanical, without insight, and usually easy to accomplish.

- Second order change involves questioning and possibly modifying deeply held personal values. These changes may deal with fundamental relationships and their modification.

First order change is directed at specific aspects that are often temporary in resolution. Second order change often results as an outgrowth or an extension of first order change. Second order change, if successful, becomes the attitude and spirit behind the action and the motivation. The goal of therapy is to attain second order change and behavior that becomes a lasting personal characteristic.

Treatment

The best method of illustrating behavioral psychotherapy as it relates to office practice is by offering examples. The following conditions are those in which some form of counseling may be required or effective, but they are by no means all inclusive. These counseling techniques can be equally effective in treating problems and modifying behavior.

Vaginismus. Patients with vaginismus can be difficult to treat if a superficial approach (reassurance only) is used.[6] In fact, many of these patients seek care from a gynecologist only to be "reassured" that they are normal (or after ill-conceived surgery for perceived abnormalities).

First Order Change

- Pelvic exam performed and normal
- Sensate focus technique
- Communication games
- Reading
- Vaginal dilatation

- Female superior intercourse
- Regular intercourse

Progression of therapy: First order change requires first meeting with the couple and allowing them to verbalize their feelings. Practitioner observation of interpersonal relationship is paramount during this initial interview. Dominant male attitude, poor self-esteem of either partner, and other therapeutic clues may become obvious. The pelvic examination should be performed to reassure the patient and practitioner that no anatomical abnormalities are present that would preclude normal penile–vaginal intercourse such as an imperforate hymen or transverse vaginal septum. The woman and man should then be separated and interviewed about sexual technique. At this time, behavior such as that demonstrated by an insensitive domineering male with no understanding of foreplay should be modified.

After the couple is reunited, the "paradox of no sexual behavior is introduced. Education and discussion of topics such as masturbation, sexual abuse, fantasies, and oral and anal sex should ensue. Educational readings should be initiated with appreciation of the patient's educational, social, and, if germane, religious background. Sensate focus techniques are begun for the female partner. The only physical interaction allowed by the couple is verbal communication. This may take place during sensate focus exercises or by writing love letters.

Small lubricated vaginal dilators are used by the patient. Once the woman is comfortable with vaginal stimulation, the male is allowed to insert a finger. The practitioner's role should be as a mediator, meeting with the couple every couple of weeks to discuss progress or problems. Progression to larger dilators, female-initiated intercourse, and finally, with permission, male-controlled intercourse is begun.

Second Order Change

After successful intercourse is established, longer-lasting issues in the relationship should be discussed. These concepts are extensions of first order changes:

- Mental/physical role reversal
- Improved communication and goals
- Orgasmic coital function

Once sexual intercourse is achieved, longer lasting goals should be determined with continued nurturing. Communications must remain a focus of the couple's relationship or sex will become purely a mechanical act. The ability to relate during the sex act (orgasmic coital function) should allow for continued communication.

Anorgasmia. Anorgasmia represents another common area of sexual therapy. Couples will usually seek care after initiating various "therapies" without understanding the fundamental physiology of female excitement. The male partner tends to be the problem partner, regardless of how well intentioned he may be.

First Order Change

- Pelvic exam to establish "normalcy"

- Sensate focus therapy
- Individual masturbation
- Mutual masturbation
- Nondemand or female-dominant coitus
- Bridging technique for sexual intercourse (face-to-face intercourse that allows manual clitoral manipulation)

Second order change should be implemented once first level change is achieved. Once the practitioner becomes comfortable with the two-stage approach to change, second order changes may be suggested during the introduction of first order, mechanical changes.

Second Order Change

- Defining the problem
- Describing attempts at solutions
- Reading assignments
- Role reversal
- "Caring days" and other relationship exercises

During therapy, the couple should see the therapist on a 2- to 3-week basis to monitor progress. The primary provider should be frank with his or her limitations; if necessary, referral to a psychiatrist earlier in the course may be in the best interest of the patient and provider.

Tobacco Abuse. Beyond the sexual aspects of counseling is behavior modification to reduce risks such as those encountered with tobacco and alcohol abuse. Cigarette abuse continues to be a major source of morbidity of women. Despite a multitude of literature and advertisements on the ill effects of cigarette use, many women continue to smoke. Many practitioners counsel their patients to quit, but without firm guidelines. By utilizing change therapy, the following scenario is possible:

First Order Change

- Nicorette gum or patches
- Group therapy
- Hypnotherapy

Second Order Change

- Increase self-esteem
- Improve self-awareness when not smoking
- Revulsion to cigarette smoke and smokers

The most important single factor in smoking cessation is patient motivation. Recurrent reminders of the health consequences of cigarette smoking may be helpful to continue motivating patients to quit. Positive reinforcement during the difficult stages of cessation by physician will be helpful in many cases.

Alcohol Abuse. Finally, another pressing problem in women's health care is alcohol use and abuse. Similar to cigarette smoking in the general population, alcohol abuse is a significant and rising health care issue. The framework for change therapy may follow the schematic outlined below.

First Order Change

- Antabuse
- Alcoholics Anonymous
- Educational group therapy
- Support groups

Once the first stages of therapy have been initiated, the patient comprehends that alcoholism is a chronic disease and failure usually results from denial that a problem exists. The second stage of therapy follows a very logical progression to second order change and, with hope, a productive and less-disruptive life.

Second Order Change

- Improve self-esteem
- Recovering of functional life-style
- Reiterate relationships
- Reestablish life goals

Trauma and High-Risk Behavior. Finally, some areas of counseling do not fit easily into the two-stage process and are purely first order change. These issues, such as accident avoidance, are mostly mechanical but represent major causes of suffering. The most important cause of morbidity and mortality in younger patients is trauma, which can be responsive to preventive measures such as the use of seat belts in automobiles. Many of the patients cared for by the obstetrician–gynecologist are young and therefore at high risk for traumatic injury, not from the sequela of chronic diseases. The use of protective helmets and equipment with cycling and other high-velocity sports should be emphasized. The newest group of orthopedic injuries is from inline skating without proper protection.

The weekend middle-aged athlete represents a growing segment of injury victims. Many attempt to participate in events that require training they lack, resulting in injuries such as ligament strains and fractures. Patients will approach the primary care physician with concerns and should be placed on a graduated exercise program with appropriate warm-up exercise and long-term goals of participation.

Continued reinforcement should be offered at visits. Infection with human immunodeficiency virus is growing in the heterosexual community at an alarming rate. Despite the heightened awareness over the past decade, even the more affluent and educated groups continue to exhibit high-risk behaviors. The practitioner should use time in contraceptive counseling of adolescent and young adults to emphasize the benefits of abstinence and safe sex behaviors. Finally, as found in other sections of this text, patients should be counseled about issues such as skin care (avoidance of ultraviolet radiation) and avoidance of disease through immunization.

Patient counseling methodology is a cornerstone of primary care in any specialty. The area of obstetrics and gynecology has many patient concerns that require sensitive and empathic counseling skills. Brief psychotherapy, with its foundations in contemporary interactional methodology, is a key component of counseling for the practicing physician. Utilizing the theories of change therapy will make brief psychotherapy relatively easy and useful, even in the busy office practice of the gynecologist.

Referral

If the practitioner does not feel comfortable with sexual counseling, then referral should be initiated. Other mental health disorders such as situational depression and neurosis may also be considered for referral depending on the interest and expertise of the individual. Disorders that are resistant to short office counseling should be recognized as soon as possible and referred to a qualified practitioner. Consultants should be screened for their willingness and expertise in dealing with women's problems. The following conditions require referral:

- Severe depression
- Bipolar mood disorders (manic–depressive personality)
- Inadequate personality disorders
- Obsessive–compulsive disorders
- Severe psychopathology (schizophrenia, etc.)

Continued observation of any of these problems or a change in behavioral patterns may be a clue that the degree of psychopathology present was underestimated during the initial assessment.

▶ REFERENCES

1. Masters WH, Johnson VE. *Human sexual inadequacy.* Boston: Little Brown, 1970.
2. Kaplan H. *The new sex therapy.* New York: Brunner/Mazel, 1974.
3. Watzlawick P, Weakland J, Fisch R. *Change: principles of problem formation and problem resolution.* New York: WW Norton, 1974.
4. Haley J. *Uncommon therapy.* New York: WW Norton, 1973.

5. *Recommendations for patient education and counseling.* United States Preventative Services Task Force. Baltimore: Williams & Wilkins, 1989, lix–lxii.
6. Fuchs K. Therapy of vaginismus by hypnotic desensitization. *Am J Obstet Gynecol* 1980;137:1–7.

CHAPTER 5

Screening: High-Risk Factors and Screening Recommendations

Between 1984 and 1988, a distinquished panel of scientists and clinicians—collectively referred to as the U.S. Public Health Task Force—met in an effort to design a framework for screening tests and preventive health care. Many of the recommendations made were collaborative and based on expert opinion but not *outcome-based* decisions. The major limitation was that many of these studies on outcome do not exist. However, in their report, the strengths and weaknesses of their recommendations were discussed and the documentation available was presented. At present, multiple studies have been designed to overcome these weaknesses and the task force is expected to release new recommendations in the next several years.

This chapter is a summary of the recommendations, which are age-group specific with special emphasis on individuals that are high risk. Throughout the text, discussion on the need for some of these schemes is debated and the controversy is addressed. Additionally, this particular area is probably the most dynamic in medicine and significant changes may be noted in the near future as better outcome studies become available. Many of the previous tenets of medicine will be challenged and, in some cases, discarded as outcome data emerge.

Some modifications to the recommendations were specific for the obstetrician–gynecologist and have been released through the American College of Obstetricians and Gynecologists in various publications. All materials found in this chapter may be found in the textbook, *Guide to Clinical Preventative Services*, published by Williams & Wilkins, Baltimore, MD, 1989.

► HIGH-RISK FACTORS

High-risk factor categories identified below are provided to focus further specific assessment and intervention where necessary. The high-risk groups described are to direct attention to detecting patients who knowingly or unknowingly fall into high-risk categories. During evaluation the patient should be made aware of high-risk conditions that require targeted screening or treatment.

> *Skin.* Persons with increased recreational or occupational exposure to sunlight, family or personal history of skin cancer, or clinical evidence of precursor lesions (e.g., dysplastic nevi, certain congenital nevi).
>
> *Hemoglobin.* Persons of Caribbean, Latin American, Asian, Mediterranean, or African descent or personal history of excessive menstrual flow.
>
> *Bacteriuria Testing.* Persons with diabetes mellitus.

STD Testing. Persons with history of multiple sexual partners, or a sexual partner with multiple contacts; sexual contacts of persons with culture-proven STD, or persons with a history of repeated episodes of STD; persons who attend clinics for sexually transmitted disease.

HIV Testing. Persons seeking treatment for sexually transmitted diseases; past or present intravenous (IV) drug users; persons with a history of prostitution; women whose past or present sexual partners were HIV infected, bisexual, or IV drug users; persons with long-term residence or birth in an area with high prevalence of HIV infection; or persons with a history of transfusion between 1978 and 1985.

Genetic Testing/Counseling. Women of reproductive age who are exposed to teratogens, or who contemplate pregnancy at age 35 or beyond. Patient, husband, or family member with history of a genetic disorder or birth defect. Persons of African–American, eastern European Jewish, Mediterranean, or Southeast Asian ancestry.

Rubella Titer/Vaccine. Females of childbearing age lacking evidence of immunity. A second measles immunization, preferably as MMR (measles–mumps–rubella vaccine), for all women unable to show proof of immunity.

Tuberculosis Skin Test. Patients infected with the human immunodeficiency virus (HIV); close contacts (sharing the same household or other enclosed environments) of persons known or suspected to have tuberculosis; persons with medical risk factors known to increase the risk of disease if infection has occurred; foreign-born persons from countries with high TB prevalence; medically underserved low-income populations; alcoholics and intravenous drug users; residents of long-term care facilities, correctional institutions, mental institutions, nursing homes/facilities, and other long-term residential facilities. Health professionals working in high-risk health care facilities.

Lipid Profile. Elevated cholesterol level, history of parent or sibling with a blood cholesterol of 240 mg/dL or higher; history of a sibling, parent, or grandparent with documented premature (age less than 55 years) coronary artery disease, presence of diabetes mellitus, or smoking habit.

Hepatitis B Vaccine. Intravenous drug users; current recipients of blood products; persons in health-related jobs with exposure to blood or blood products; household and sexual contacts with HBV carriers, sexually active persons with multiple sexual partners diagnosed as having recently acquired sexually transmitted diseases, prostitutes and persons who have a history of sexual activity with multiple partners in the previous 6 months.

Fluoride Supplement. Persons living in areas with inadequate water fluoridation (less than 0.7 parts/million).

Mammogram. Women age 35 and older with a family history of premenopausally diagnosed breast cancer in a first-degree relative.

Fasting Glucose Test. Every 3–5 years if family history (one first-degree or two second-degree relatives) of diabetes mellitus; or if markedly obese or personal history of gestational diabetes mellitus. (Cutoff is 140 mg/dL.)

Thyroid-Stimulating Hormone. Individuals with a strong family history of thyroid disease, and patients with autoimmune diseases. There is some evidence that subclinical hypothyroidism may be related to unfavorable lipid profiles.

Influenza Vaccine. Residents of chronic care facilities and persons suffering from chronic cardiopulmonary disorders, metabolic diseases including diabetes, hemoglobinopathies, immunosuppression, or renal dysfunction.

Pneumococcal Vaccine. Persons with medical conditions that increase the risk of pneumococcal infection (e.g., chronic cardiac or pulmonary disease, sickle cell disease, nephrotic syndrome, Hodgkin's disease, asplenia, diabetes, alcoholism, cirrhosis, multiple myeloma, renal disease, or other immunosuppression).

Colonoscopy. Persons with a personal history of inflammatory bowel disease or colonic polyps; or family history of familial polyposis coli, colorectal cancer, or cancer family syndrome. In addition to high-risk factors related to each age group, the physician should be aware of the Leading Causes of Death and Leading Causes of Morbidity of women by age group. The perspective added by the recognition of these causes enhances the overall approach to the patient's continuing care.

▶ AGES 12 YEARS AND UNDER

For this age group, the obstetrician–gynecologist functions as a consultant only. It is anticipated that most patients in this age category will be under the care of a specialist in pediatrics or a specialist in family medicine. Therefore, the screening necessary for all children should be done by that physician. The obstetrician–gynecologist usually serves in the capacity of a consultant and any tests or evaluation performed would most likely be toward a diagnosis, not screening.

► AGES 13–18

(Schedule: Yearly, or as appropriate)

1. Obtain responses to Patient Questionnaire.
2. Review Problem List and Continuity of Care Records.

Screening

Periodic History

a) Health status, medical, surgical, family
b) Elaboration of presenting complaint, if any
c) Dietary/nutritional assessment
d) Physical activity
e) Tobacco, alcohol, drug use
f) Abuse/neglect
g) Sexual practices

Periodic Physical

a) Height
b) Weight
c) Blood pressure
d) Secondary sexual characteristics (Tanner Staging)
e) Pelvic examination: yearly when sexually active, or by age 18
f) Skin

Laboratory

a) PAP test: yearly when sexually active, or by age 18

High-Risk Group

a) Hemoglobin
b) Bacteriuria testing
c) STD testing
d) HIV testing
e) Genetic testing/counseling
f) Rubella titer
g) Tuberculosis skin test
h) Lipid profile

Evaluation and Counseling

Sexuality

a) Development
b) High-risk behaviors
c) Contraceptive options
Genetic counseling
Prevention of unwanted pregnancy
d) Sexually transmitted diseases
Partner selection
Barrier protection

Fitness

a) Hygiene (including dental)
b) Dietary/nutritional assessment
c) Exercise: selection of program

Psychosocial

a) Interpersonal/family relationships

b) Sexual identity

c) Personal goal development

d) Behavioral/learning disorders

e) Abuse/neglect

Cardiovascular Risk Factors

a) Family history

b) Hypertension

c) Hyperlipidemia

d) Obesity/diabetes

Health/Risk Behaviors

a) Injury prevention
  Safety belts/safety helmets
  Recreational hazards
  Firearms
  Hearing

b) Skin exposure to ultraviolet rays

c) Suicide–depressive symptoms

d) Tobacco, alcohol, other drugs

Immunizations

Immunizations

a) Tetanus–diphtheria booster: once between ages 14 and 16

High-Risk Groups

a) Measles–mumps–rubella (MMR)
b) Hepatitis B vaccine
e) Fluoride supplement

Leading Causes of Death	Leading Causes of Morbidity
Motor vehicle accidents	Nose, throat, and upper respiratory infections
Homicide, suicide	
Leukemia	Viral, bacterial, and parasitic diseases
Injuries (musculoskeletal and soft tissue)	
	Sexual abuse
	Acute ear infections
	Digestive system conditions
	Acute urinary conditions

▶ AGES 19–39

(Schedule: Yearly, or as appropriate)

1. Obtain responses to Patient Questionnaire.
2. Review Problem List and Continuity of Care Records.

Screening

Periodic History

a) Health status, medical, surgical, family
b) Elaboration of presenting complaint, if any

c) Dietary/nutritional assessment

d) Physical activity

e) Tobacco, alcohol, drug use

f) Abuse/neglect

g) Sexual practices

Periodic Physical

a) Height

b) Weight

c) Blood pressure

d) Neck: adenopathy, thyroid

e) Breasts

f) Abdomen

g) Pelvic examination

h) Skin

Laboratory

a) Pap test: physician and patient discretion after three consecutive normal tests

b) Cholesterol: every 5 years

High-Risk Groups

a) Hemoglobin

b) Bacteriuria testing

c) Mammogram

d) Fasting glucose test

e) STD testing
f) HIV testing
g) Genetic testing/counseling
h) Tuberculosis skin test
i) Lipid profile
j) Thyroid-stimulating hormone

Evaluation and Counseling

Sexuality

a) High-risk behaviors
b) Contraceptive options
   Genetic counseling
   Prevention of unwanted pregnancy
c) Sexually transmitted disease
   Partner selection
   Barrier protection
d) Sexual functioning

Fitness

a) Hygiene (including dental)
b) Dietary/nutritional assessment
c) Exercise: selection of program

Psychosocial

a) Interpersonal/family relationships
b) Domestic violence

c) Job satisfaction

d) Life-style/stress

e) Sleep disorders

Cardiovascular Risk Factors

a) Family history

b) Hypertension

c) Hyperlipidemia

d) Obesity/diabetes

e) Life-style

Health/Risk Behaviors

a) Injury prevention
Safety belts/safety helmets
Occupational hazards
Recreational hazards
Firearms
Hearing

b) Breast self-examination

c) Skin exposure to ultraviolet rays

d) Suicide–depressive symptoms

e) Tobacco, alcohol, other drugs

Immunizations

Immunizations

a) Tetanus–diphtheria booster every 10 years

High-Risk Groups

a) Measles–mumps–rubella (MMR)

b) Hepatitis B vaccine

c) Influenza vaccine

d) Pneumococcal vaccine

Leading Causes of Death	Leading Causes of Morbidity
Motor vehicle accidents	Nose, throat, and upper respiratory infections
Cardiovascular disease	
Homicide	Injuries (musculoskeletal and soft tissue, (including back and upper and lower extremities)
Coronary artery disease	
AIDS	
Breast cancer	Viral, bacterial, and parasitic diseases
Cerebrovascular disease	
Uterine cancer	Acute urinary conditions

▶ AGES 40–64

(Schedule: Yearly, or as appropriate)

1. Obtain responses to Patient Questionnaire.

2. Review Problem List and Continuity of Care Records.

Screening

Periodic History

a) Health status, medical, surgical, family

b) Elaboration of presenting complaint, if any

c) Dietary/nutritional assessment

d) Physical activity

e) Tobacco, alcohol, drug use

f) Abuse/neglect

g) Sexual practices

Periodic Physical

a) Height

b) Weight

c) Blood pressure

d) Oral cavity

e) Neck: adenopathy, thyroid

f) Breasts, axillae

g) Abdomen

h) Pelvic and rectovaginal examination

i) Skin

Laboratory

a) Pap test: physician and patient discretion after three consecutive normal tests

b) Mammogram: every 1–2 years until age 50, yearly beginning at age 50

c) Cholesterol: every 5 years

d) Fecal occult blood test

e) Sigmoidoscopy: after age 50, every 3–5 years

High-Risk Groups

a) Hemoglobin

b) Bacteriuria testing

c) Mammogram

d) Fasting glucose test

e) STD testing

f) HIV testing

g) Tuberculosis skin test

h) Lipid profile

i) Thyroid-stimulating hormone

j) Colonoscopy

Evaluation and Counseling

Sexuality

a) High-risk behaviors

b) Contraceptive options
Genetic counseling
Prevention of unwanted pregnancy

c) Sexually transmitted disease
Partner selection
Barrier protection

d) Sexual functioning

Fitness

a) Hygiene (including dental)
b) Dietary/nutritional assessment
c) Exercise: selection of program

Psychosocial Evaluation

a) Family relationships
b) Domestic violence
c) Job/work satisfaction
d) Retirement planning
e) Life-style/stress
f) Sleep disorders

Cardiovascular Risk Factors

a) Family history
b) Hypertension
c) Hyperlipidemia
d) Obesity/diabetes
e) Life-style

Health/Risk Behaviors

a) Hormone replacement therapy
b) Injury prevention
    Safety belts/safety helmets
    Occupational hazards
    Recreational hazards
    Sports involvement
    Firearms
    Hearing

c) Breast self-examination

d) Skin exposure to ultraviolet rays

e) Suicide–depressive symptoms

f) Tobacco, alcohol, other drugs

Immunizations

Immunizations

a) Tetanus–diphtheria booster: every 10 years

b) Influenza vaccine: annually beginning at age 55

High-Risk Groups

a) Measles–mumps–rubella

b) Hepatitis B vaccine

c) Influenza vaccine

d) Pneumococcal vaccine

Leading Causes of Death	Leading Causes of Morbidity
Cardiovascular disease	Nose, throat, and upper respiratory infections
Coronary artery disease	
Breast cancer	Osteoporosis/arthritis
Lung cancer	Hypertension
Cerebrovascular disease	Orthopedic deformities and impairments (including back and upper and lower extremities)
Colorectal cancer	
Heart disease	
Obstructive pulmonary disease	Hearing and vision impairments
Ovarian cancer	

▶ AGES 65 YEARS AND OLDER

(Schedule: Yearly, or as appropriate)

1.   Obtain responses to Patient Questionnaire.
2.   Review Problem List and Continuity of Care Records.

Screening

Periodic History

a)   Health status, medical, surgical, family
b)   Elaboration of presenting complaint, if any
c)   Dietary/nutritional assessment
d)   Physical activity
e)   Tobacco, alcohol, drug use, polypharmacy
f)   Abuse/neglect
g)   Sexual practices

Periodic Physical

a)   Height
b)   Weight
c)   Blood pressure
d)   Oral cavity
e)   Neck: adenopathy, thyroid
f)   Breasts, axillae
g)   Abdomen

h) Pelvic and rectovaginal examination

i) Skin

Laboratory

a) Pap test: physician and patient discretion after three consecutive normal tests

b) Urinalysis/dipstick

c) Mammogram

d) Cholesterol: every 3–5 years

e) Fecal occult blood test

f) Sigmoidoscopy: every 3–5 years

g) Thyroid-stimulating hormone test: every 3–5 years

High-Risk Groups

a) Hemoglobin

b) Fasting glucose test

c) STD testing

d) HIV testing

e) Tuberculosis skin test

f) Lipid profile

g) Colonoscopy

Evaluation and Counseling

Sexuality

a) Sexual functioning

b) Sexual behaviors

c) Sexually transmitted diseases

Fitness

a) Hygiene (general and dental)

b) Dietary/nutritional assessment

c) Exercise: selection of program

Psychosocial Evaluation

a) Neglect/abuse

b) Life-style/stress

c) Depression/sleep disorders

d) Family relationships

e) Job/work/retirement satisfaction

Cardiovascular Risk Factors

a) Hypertension

b) Hypercholesterolemia

c) Obesity/diabetes

d) Sedentary life-style

Health/Risk Behaviors

a) Hormone replacement therapy

b) Injury prevention
Safety belts/safety helmets

Occupational hazards

Recreational hazards

Hearing

Firearms

c) Visual acuity/glaucoma

d) Hearing

e) Breast self-examination

f) Skin exposure to ultraviolet rays

g) Suicide–depressive symptoms

h) Tobacco, alcohol, other drugs

Immunizations

Immunizations

a) Tetanus–diphtheria booster: every 10 years

b) Influenza vaccine: annually

c) Pneumococcal vaccine: Once

High-Risk Groups

a) Hepatitis B vaccine

Leading Causes of Death	Leading Causes of Morbidity
Cardiovascular disease	Nose, throat, and upper respiratory infections
Coronary artery disease	
Cerebrovascular disease	Osteoporosis/arthritis
Pneumonia/influenza	Hypertension
Obstructive lung disease	Urinary incontinence
Colorectal cancer	Heart disease
Breast cancer	Injuries (musculoskeletal and soft tissue)
Hearing and vision impairments	
Lung cancer	
Accident	

CARDIOVASCULAR AND LIPID DISEASES

Cardiovascular disease usually occurs secondary to four major disease conditions: hypertension, diabetes mellitus, hypercholesterolemia, and tobacco addiction. Chapter 6 is devoted to the diagnosis and control of hypertension. Hypertension, which is more common in women than men over the age of 50, has a direct effect on vascular endothelium that contributes to atherosclerotic plaque formation. Large epidemiologic studies have demonstrated that minimal decreases in systolic and diastolic blood pressures can make a significant difference in the prevention of cardiovascular disease, especially coronary artery disease and stroke. Although it was once thought that control of diastolic blood pressure was the only important facet of disease prevention, recent studies of hypertension have focused on the role of systolic blood pressure as a key independent variable. Additionally, the long-term effect of hypertension on ventricle wall thickness has been appreciated as an important risk factor for

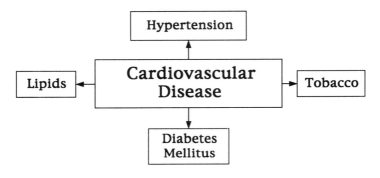

stroke. Life-style modifications such as exercise, cigarette smoking cessation, low sodium diet, weight control, and reduction of alcohol intake are now first-line therapy in mild hypertension.

Cardiovascular disease is not directly related to just a single risk factor but rather is a global disease with many contributing factors such as family history, diabetes, and dyslipidemias. Chapter 7 will deal with lipids and Chapter 8 in the next section will deal with diabetes. Targeting risk factors and their modification are important aspects of therapy—younger individuals with several risk factors may be more aggressively treated than individuals with no risk factors. Therefore, diabetes and hypercholesterolemia must play a central role in any discussion of cardiovascular disease. Finally, risk factors for cardiac disease should be noted and quantified on the patient's chart.

Risk Factors for Coronary Heart Disease

Positive Predictors

- Male: Age > 45 years
- Female: Age > 55 years
  No estrogen replacement therapy (ERT)
  Pemature menopause without ERT
- Cigarette smoking
- Hypertension (blood pressure of >140/90 or on treatment)
- Diabetes
- HDL-cholesterol < 35 mg/dL
- Family history of myocardial infarction or sudden death prior to 55 years in first-degree male relative, or 65 in first-degree female relative

Negative Risk Factor

- HDL-cholesterol > 60 mg/dL (also allows subtraction of one risk factor)

Adapted from National Institutes of Health Publication 93-3095. Second report of the expert panel on detection, evaluation, and treatment of high blood cholesterol in adults. Page I-11.

CHAPTER 6

Hypertension

Hypertension contributes significantly to morbidity and mortality in women. After age 50, women have a higher incidence of hypertension than men. Between the ages of 65 and 74, an estimated 65% of women are affected. There is a firmly established relationship between hypertension and cardiovascular events such as stroke, coronary artery disease, congestive heart disease, and renal disease. Genetic factors have not been well characterized; however, hypertension occurs twice as often in African–Americans than it does in whites. Hypertension is defined as a systolic pressure greater than 140 and a diastolic pressure greater than 90 on two separate occasions. A classification of hypertension is shown in Table 6-1.

Screening

Blood pressure should be determined at each office visit. In the evaluation of hypertension, measurement technique is an essential variable to control. "White coat" or factitious office hypertension exists in up to 30% of patients and may be population dependent.[1] Ambulatory monitoring or home monitoring is worthwhile in many cases, especially if this influence is suspected. Blood pressure has a diurnal pattern (highest at

▶ **TABLE 6-1   Classification of Hypertension**

Category	Systolic (mm Hg)	Diastolic (mm Hg)
Normal	<130	<85
High normal	130–139	85– 89
Hypertension[a]		
Stage 1 (mild)	140–159	90– 99
Stage 2 (moderate)	160–179	100–109
Stage 3 (severe)	180–209	110–119
Stage 4 (very severe)	≥210	≥120

[a]Based on the aveage of two or more readings taken at two or more visits after an initial screening.

Source: Joint National Committee on the Detection, Evaluation, and Treatment of High Blood Pressure. *Arch Intern Med* 1993;153:154–83.

mid-day and lowest between midnight and 4 am), so determinations should be performed at the same time of day.

Blood pressure should be measured after the patient has rested for 5 minutes in a seated position. The right arm is preferred because blood pressure is higher in that arm. Cuff placement and cuff size are important variables (Table 6-2). Most blood pressure cuffs are marked with "normal limits." The most commonly encountered error in the measurement of blood pressure is the use of a cuff that is too small on an obese patient, resulting in falsely high blood pressure or "cuff hypertension." The cuff should be applied 2 cm above the bend of the elbow with the arm positioned parallel to the floor. The cuff should be inflated to 30 mm Hg beyond the point of the disappearance of the brachial pulse, or 220 mm Hg. The cuff should be deflated slowly at a rate of no more than 2 mm Hg/second.[2]

There is controversy regarding the interpretation of diastolic blood pressure measurements performed with a stetho-

► TABLE 6-2   Common Errors in Measuring Blood Pressure

	Effect on Blood Pressure	
Error	Falsely High	Falsely Low
Blood pressure cuff		
Too narrow	✓	
Wrapped too loosely	✓	
Deflated too slowly	✓	
Korotkoff's sounds		
Difficult to hear	✓ (diastolic)	✓ (systolic)
Cuff released too rapidly	✓	✓
(>2 mm Hg/seconds)	(diastolic)	(systolic)
Arm relationship to heart level		
Above it		✓
Below it	✓	

Source: Nolan TE. Evaluation and treatment of uncomplicated hypertension in the gynecologic patient. *Female Patient* 1992;17:13–21.

scope. Phase IV Korotkoff's sounds are described as the point when pulsations are muffled, whereas phase V occurs when all sound disappears. Most experts in the management of hypertension advocate the use of phase V Korotkoff's sounds as a means of assessing diastolic blood pressure. Regardless of the method used, repeated measurements should be performed with a 2-minute rest between readings, and two measurements with less than a 10 mm Hg difference should be obtained.

Automated devices have helped standardize measurements but they are not perfect and readings should be correlated with other techniques of measurement. Two types of automated sphygmomanometers are readily available for home monitoring: (1) *auscultatory,* which uses a small microphone placed over the brachial artery, or (2) *oscillometry,* which measures fluctuations of brachial artery pulsations. Regardless of the type of device used, patients should demonstrate their ability to use the equipment while they are in the office. Office readings should be correlated with the home device. Certain patients, particularly those who are anxious and/or not highly motivated, may not be good candidates for home monitoring.

Following are key historical factors that should be determined in the initial history:

- Prior recognition of high blood pressure readings (how often, when, and if evaluated)
- Prior use of any antihypertensive medications
- Other medical complicating factors (i.e., headaches, myocardial infarction or chest pain, prior stroke, evidence of renal disease)
- Excessive sodium or alcohol use or special diets or medications (i.e., adrenocorticosteroids and sympathomimetics and nasal decongestants).
- Other cardiovascular risk factors, including pack years of smoking, cholesterol measurements, obesity, and diabetes mellitus
- Family history of cardiovascular disease prior to age 55 in parents or siblings, as well as the cause and age of death.

Baseline laboratory evaluations are recommended in the initial evaluation of patients with hypertension to rule out secondary forms or reversible causes of hypertension:

- Dipstick urinalysis (microscopic indicated if any values abnormal)

- Creatinine, potassium, fasting glucose concentration
- Total cholesterol, HDL-cholesterol, and fasting trigly-cerides
- Electrocardiogram

If the patient has other cardiovascular disease or target organ disease, referral is indicated.

Treatment

An approach to management is outlined in Figure 6-1. The first step in treatment of patients with mild and moderate hypertension is life-style modification[3]:

- Weight reduction if the patient is overweight
- Limitation of alcohol use to <1 ounce of absolute alcohol (2 beers, 8 ounces of wine, 2 ounces of 100 proof whiskey)
- Aerobic exercise (30 minutes fast walking 3 times/week)
- Limitation of salt intake to less than 6 grams daily
- Smoking cessation
- Limitation of dietary saturated fats and cholesterol
- Adequate intake of calcium, potassium, and magnesium
- Glucose control for patients with diabetes

The effectiveness of these interventions should be strictly observed over a 3- to 6-month period. Blood pressure readings should be obtained frequently either by an ambulatory device, in the office two to four times a month, or by a qualified nurse. If life-style modification is successful, monitoring should continue at 3–6-month intervals for 1–2 years (Table 6-3). When

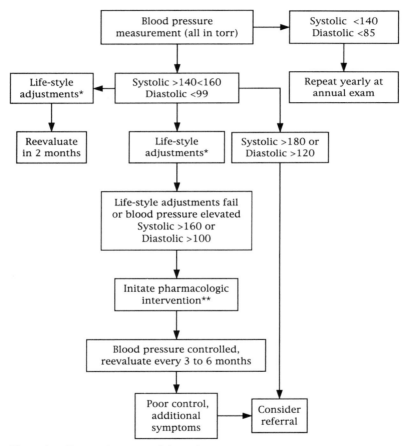

*Excercise, dietary changes, weight and alcohol reduction.
** See Table 6-4

FIGURE 6-1. Algorithm for the management of essential hypertension.

▶ **TABLE 6-3   Recommended Intervals for Follow-up**

Systolic (mm Hg)	Diastolic (mm Hg)	Follow-up Recommendation
<130	85	Recheck in 2 years
130–139	85–89	Recheck in 1 year, diet, etc.
140–159	90–99	Confirm in 2 months
160–179	100–109	Evaluate or refer in 1 month
180–209	110–119	Evaluate or refer in 1 week
≥210	≥120	Refer immediately

Source: Joint National Committee on the Detection, Evaluation, and Treatment of High Blood Pressure. *Arch Intern Med* 1993;153:154–83.

life-style modification is not successful, medication should be given to decrease target organ disease.

Concurrent medical conditions and racial characteristics may influence treatment options. Migraine headache sufferers are best treated with beta-blocking agents or calcium channel agonists. African–Americans may respond less well to beta blockers or angiotensin-converting enzyme (ACE) inhibitors and best to diuretics and calcium channel blockers.[4]

Patients who can monitor their blood pressure at home should measure and record their blood pressure twice weekly. When medications are started, a follow-up assessment should be scheduled in 2–4 weeks. Effectiveness of therapy and side effect profiles should be determined. Single agents improve compliance; if initial doses are ineffective, the dosage should be increased. If the medication is ineffective or side effects develop, a different class of drug may be used or a second drug could be added. The goal of therapy is to lower blood pressure into the normal range (a systolic level of <140 mm Hg and a diastolic level of <85 mm Hg). The number of antihyperten-

► **TABLE 6-4 Selected Medications and Dosages for Control of Essential Hypertension**

Medication (Class)	Normal Daily Dosage (mg/day) and Interval	Dispensing Unit
Angiotensin-converting enzyme (ACE) inhibitors		
Enalapril	5–40 (qd, bid)	2.5, 5, 10, 20
Calcium channel blockers		
Nifedipine sustained release	30–90 (qd)	30, 60, 90
Diltiazem sustained release	120–240 (bid)	60, 90, 120
Alpha-blockers		
Terazosin	1–20 (qd)	1, 2, 5, 10
Mixed Alpha- and Beta-blockers		
Labetalol	200–800 (bid)	100, 200, 300
Diuretics		
Hydrochlorothiazide	12.5–50 (qd)	25, 50
Triamterene (potassium-sparing)	50–100 (bid)	50, 100
Beta-blockers		
Propranolol (lipid soluble)	60–160 (qd)	60, 80, 120, 160
Atenolol (water soluble)	50–100 (qd)	50, 100
Smooth muscle relaxant		
Hydralazine	25–75 (tid, qid)	10, 25, 50, 100

sive agents available has exploded over the past decade, and common dosages are found in Table 6-4.

In the past, therapy was instituted in steps, starting with thiazides, followed by the addition of beta-blocking agents, and finally followed by vasodilator drugs. The newer drugs (ACE inhibitors, postadrenergic ganglionic blocking agents, and calcium channel-blocking agents) are more potent, have longer half-lives, and are useful as single agents.

Diuretics. Until the past 10 years, the most commonly used medication had been the thiazide diuretics. Despite the introduction of newer therapeutic classes of drugs that have fewer side effects and better blood pressure-lowering characteristics, thiazide diuretics are still useful in some cases. Recent evidence suggests that the maximum therapeutic dose of thiazide should be 25 mg rather than the 50 mg previously used. Potassium-sparing diuretics (spironolactone, triamterene, or amiloride) are more effective than supplementation to maintain potassium levels and should be prescribed to prevent the development of hypokalemia. Thiazide diuretics cause hyperuricemia and may contribute to acute gout attacks. They also can cause glucose intolerance and hyperlipidemia.[5] These side effects have recently led many experts to question the widespread use of these drugs.

Angiotensin-Converting Enzyme Inhibitors. Angiotensin-converting enzyme inhibitors have quickly become a first-line drug in hypertensive therapy. These drugs are relatively safe and have few side effects (occasional hypotension with the first dose, blood dyscrasias, and a chronic cough) and rarely interfere with quality of life. Because ACE inhibitors have adverse effects during gestation, other agents should be considered for patients who potentially could be pregnant. They can be used successfully with other agents including diuretics, beta-blocking agents, and calcium channel agonists. Unlike beta-blocking agents, ACE inhibitors can be used for patients who have asthma, chronic obstructive airway disease, depression, diabetes, and peripheral vascular disease. Multiple formulations introduced in the past 5 years have long half-lives, resulting in daily dosing and thus increased popularity as first-line therapy. Occasionally, patients will suffer from rashes, loss of taste, fatigue, and headaches. As a class, ACE inhibitors are less effective in African–Americans than in other populations unless they are used in combination with a diuretic.

Beta-Blocking Agents. Beta-blocking agents have been used extensively for over 20 years as antihypertensive drugs. As a class, they are an excellent source of first-line therapy, especially for patients who suffer from migraine headaches. The original formulation, propranolol, was highly lipid soluble, which resulted in many side effects such as depression, sleep disturbances (nightmares in the elderly), and constipation. Additionally, it was not beta select (propranolol has both beta$_1$ and beta$_2$ effects), leading to more side effects. The newer formulations (e.g., atenolol) are water soluble and beta$_1$ selective and thus have fewer side effects. They also have longer half-lives than lipid-soluble preparations and can be given in single daily doses, which increases compliance. These drugs have a negative impact on cholesterol levels and thus should be avoided in patients who have hyperlipidemia. Contraindications to the use of beta-blocking agents are asthma, chronic obstructive pulmonary diseases, congestive heart failure, and sick sinus syndrome. These agents should not be discontinued acutely in patients who have angina because a *rebound phenomenon* of ischemia may precipitate an acute myocardial infarction. Despite these limitations, beta-blocking agents continue to be useful, especially for counteracting the reflex tachycardia that occurs with the use of smooth muscle-relaxing drugs (e.g., hydralazine).

Vasodilators. Hydralazine is a vasodilator whose mechanism of action is direct relaxation of arterial wall smooth muscle. Major side effects are headache, tachycardia, and fluid retention. The addition of a beta-blocking agent limits tachycardia and headaches without compromising the blood pressure-lowering effects. Drug-induced lupus is a well-recognized side effect, but it is rare at normal therapeutic doses (25–50 mg three times daily). Minoxidil is another commonly used drug in this class, but it is of limited use in women because it increases beard growth.

Alpha₁-Adrenergic Drugs. Alpha₁-adrenergic drugs have become popular because of their unique relationship to lipids. When these drugs are used as single agents, total cholesterol and low-density lipoprotein decrease while high-density lipoprotein increases. The mode of action is the blockage of postganglionic norepinephrine vasoconstriction in peripheral vascular smooth muscle. Prazosin and doxazosin are the most popular preparations available in this group. A serious side effect is the "first-dose effect" when severe orthostasis can occur in some patients, most commonly the elderly. Patients should be instructed to begin use with a small dose at bedtime for several days prior to increasing dosage or changing dosing schedules. Other side effects include tachycardia, weakness, dizziness, and mild fluid retention. Because of the alpha-blocking effect on the urethra, it may produce stress urinary incontinence in women with borderline sphincter control mechanisms.[6]

Calcium Channel-Blocking Agents. Calcium channel-blocking agents have been a major therapeutic breakthrough for patients with coronary artery disease. As a secondary effect, they are effective for the control of peripheral vascular disease and hypertension. Patients whose condition is difficult to control, such as the elderly and African–Americans, respond well to this class of medications. These drugs also are highly effective in treating concurrent angina and migraine headache. Long-acting calcium channel-blocking agents allow medication to be given in a single dose, resulting in wide acceptance of therapy.

Central-Acting Agents. Central-acting agents (i.e., methyldopa and clonidine) have been used for decades, especially in obstetrics. Side effects, including taste disorders, dry mouth, and need for frequent dosing (except for the transdermal form of clonidine), have limited the popularity of these drugs. Compliance is a major issue for all medications, and as new classes of drugs are introduced, the use of this class of drugs will probably continue to decline.

Referral

Abnormal laboratory values may indicate secondary causes of hypertension, which require more extensive evaluations and possibly surgery. The following patients should be referred to the appropriate specialist for more intensive therapy and monitoring:

- Patients with markedly elevated systolic or diastolic pressure (e.g., systolic > 160 mm Hg and diastolic > 110 mm Hg)
- Patients who do not respond to single-agent therapy or who have other diseases (i.e., coronary artery disease, diabetes mellitus, peripheral vascular disease)

- Patients whose condition is resistant to therapy who may have unrecognized early end-stage disease
- Patients with evidence of target organ disease

▶ REFERENCES

1. Julius S, Mejia A, Jones K, et al. "White coat" versus "sustained" borderline hypertension in Tecumseh, Michigan. *Hypertension* 1990;16:617–23.

2. American Society of Hypertension. Recommendations for routine blood pressure measurement by indirect cuff sphygmomanometry. *Am J Hypertens* 1992;5:207–9.

3. Stamler R, Stamler J, Grimm R, et al. Nutritional therapy for high blood pressure: final report of a four-year randomized controlled trial—the Hypertension Control Program. *JAMA* 1987;257:1484–91.

4. Moorman PG, Hames CG, Tyroler HA. Socioeconomic status and morbidity and mortality in hypertensive blacks. *Cardiovasc Clin* 1991;21(3):179–94.

5. Freis ED. Critique of the clinical importance of diuretic-induced hypokalemia and elevated cholesterol level. *Arch Intern Med* 1989;149:2640–8.

6. Dwyer PL, Teele JS. Prazosin: a neglected cause of genuine stress incontinence. *Obstet Gynecol* 1992;79:117–21.

CHAPTER 7

Cholesterol

► HISTORY AND DIAGNOSIS

Cholesterol metabolism, despite popular discussion, is not determined exclusively by LDL- and HDL-cholesterol but by various protein carriers with receptors in different tissues. Cholesterol is usually found in an esterized form with various proteins and glycerides, which define the metabolic step. The following components are important lipid particles in cholesterol metabolism.

Lipid Particles

Chylomicrons are large lipoprotein particles made of dietary triglycerides and cholesterol. Chylomicrons are prehepatic and secreted in the intestinal lumen, are absorbed in the lymph, and then pass into the general circulation. They may be used in adipose tissue and skeletal muscle for energy production. Lipoprotein particles are formed from three major components. The core consists of triglycerides and cholesterol esters in varying amounts depending on the stage of the metabolic pathway. Surrounding the nonpolar core is a surface coat of *apoproteins* and structural proteins.

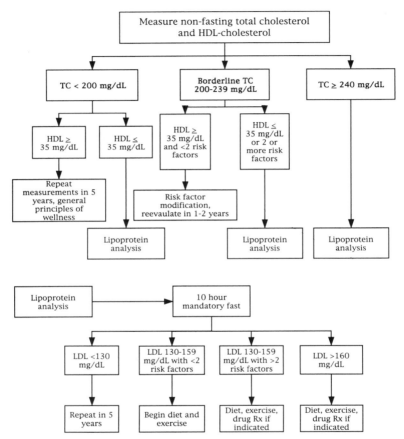

FIGURE 7-1. Management scheme for measurement and therapy of increased levels of cholesterol. TC, total cholesterol; LDL, LDL-cholesterol; HDL, HDL-cholesterol. Adapted from Second report of the expert panel on detection, evaluation, and treatment of high blood cholesterol in adults. NIH Publication 93-3095, 1993.

Apoproteins (apo) are specific recognition proteins exposed at the surface of a lipoprotein particle. Certain apoproteins are associated with specific types of cholesterol, for example, apoprotein A-I and apoprotein A-II are associated with HDL-cholesterol, the so-called scavenger cholesterol. Apoprotein C-II has additional activity as a cofactor for lipoprotein lipase. Mutated apoproteins are currently identified as markers for premature atherosclerosis and in the future may be more predictive of premature cardiovascular disease then LDL- and HDL-cholesterol.

Subdivisions of the lipoprotein classes are described below and summarized in Figure 7-1.

Prehepatic Metabolites. *Chylomicrons and remnants* are composed of major lipids and apoproteins of the A, B-48, C, and E classes. These are large particles synthesized from dietary cholesterols and absorbed triglycerides. Elevated levels of these components may be significant indicators of atherosclerosis and may explain differences in individuals in the development of atherosclerosis.

Posthepatic Metabolites. *VLDLs* (very-low-density lipoproteins) are transient remnants from initial liver metabolism and compose only 10–15% of cholesterol particles. VLDLs consist of endogenously synthesized triglycerides. *IDLs* (intermediate density lipoproteins) are lipids that consist of cholesterol esters and are posthepatic remnants. Apoprotein B-48 is lost after the initial hepatic metabolism and B-100 is substituted. Apo E, which is a liver recognition apoprotein, is found only in VLDL and IDL. Various combinations of alleles from apo E are also associated with atherosclerosis. IDL metabolites are transient lipoproteins, measured only in certain pathological conditions.

The major lipid in the *LDL*-cholesterol group is the cholesterol ester and is associated with B-100 apoprotein. LDL-cholesterol is approximately 60–70% of total cholesterol. Elevated levels of LDL-cholesterol have been associated with increased myocardial infarction in women over 65 years of age. Several families have been described with structurally abnormal B-100 apoprotein and are at high risk for myocardial infarction due to lipid buildup and premature atherosclerosis.[1] Density ranges from 1.019 to 1.063, with a diameter of 180–280 nm.

HDL-cholesterol is composed of cholesterol esters with apoproteins A-I and A-II. These particles are 20–30% of total cholesterol and are the most dense with a weight of 1.063–1.120 g/mL. The diameter of this group of proteins is 50–120 nm.

Lipoprotein [a] or Lp[a] is an inherited lipoprotein. High levels are associated with elevated triglycerides, elevated LDL-cholesterol, and low HDL-cholesterol. High levels have been associated with myocardial infarction.[2,3] Estrogen and cyclic progesterone replacement therapy decreases Lp[a], triglycerides, and LDL-cholesterol and increases HDL-cholesterol, suggesting a mechanism for delayed atherosclerosis and cardiovascular death in women.[4]

Cholesterol metabolism is divided into two pathways: the *exogenous* pathway derived from *dietary* sources and the *endogenous pathway* or the *lipid transport pathway*. Individual variations exist in the ability to metabolize cholesterol: normals, hypo-responders, and hyper-responders.[5] Early evidence suggests that some individuals will respond to diet, others to certain drugs, and some to neither. These may be explained by genetic differences in apo E recognition factors. Hypo-responders may be given cholesterol-loaded diets with no effect on serum cholesterol measurement. The hyper-responder, in contrast, has a high serum cholesterol, regardless of dietary intake. Explanations of why these differences exist are well described in animal models but not in humans. A graphic representation of the metabolic routes is found in Figure 7-2. Further explanation is beyond the scope of this discussion.

When cholesterol is measured, various fractions are reported. Plasma cholesterol or *total cholesterol* consists of cholesteryl and unesterified cholesterol fractions. If triglycerides are analyzed in conjunction with cholesterol, then assumptions can be made concerning which metabolic pathway may be abnormal. If both total cholesterol and triglycerides are elevated, this signifies a problem with chylomicrons and VLDL synthesis. If the triglyceride/cholesterol ratio is greater than 5:1, then the predominant fractions are chylomicrons and VLDLs. When the triglyceride/cholesterol ratio is less than 5:1, then the problem exists in the VLDL and LDL fractions. Hyperlipoproteinemias are defined by establishing a "normal population" and then setting various limits at the 10th and 90th percentiles. Recent standards for women set the 80th percentile for cholesterol at 240 mg/dL and the 50th percentile at 200 mg/dL. Researchers continue to argue that the population being studied may have different cutoff limits depending on the amount of fat versus vegetable and fiber consumption within the diet.[6]

Plasma elevations of chylomicrons, LDLs, VLDLs, various remnants of IDLs, and VLDLs and chylomicrons are classified by the elevated fraction. This adds to the confusion of an already difficult topic. Unfortunately, this classifi-

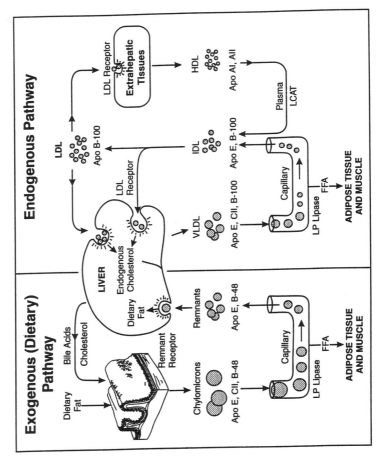

FIGURE 7-2. A graphic representation of the metabolic routes.

cation of hyperlipoproteinemias is the basis of studying disease states.

Screening

In the past decade, cholesterol testing has become something of a fad. Stratification of high- and low-risk groups for screening may help to eliminate unnecessary testing. Even though some groups suggest cholesterol testing begin after 20 years of age and continue every 5 years to the menopause, there are few data to support testing in low-risk women. After age 65, testing is increased to every 3 years. High-risk groups include those with the following characteristics:

- Family history of cardiovascular events prior to age 55
- Hypertension
- Cigarette smoking
- Obesity ($>$120% of normal weight)
- Diabetes
- Menopause (regardless of type) without hormonal replacement therapy
- Hypothyroidism

The United States Preventative Services Task Force recommends testing (on the basis of expert opinion, but not on epidemiological data) every 5 years beginning in the 19–39-year-old age group and continuing through life. As previously stated, this may represent overtesting, and the clinician should judge appropriate intervals in the treating population.

Office laboratory analyzers of total cholesterol are inaccurate because techniques for measurement and standardization are difficult to maintain. In well-controlled studies, variation in readings is large.[7] There are multiple environmental causes of variation in cholesterol measurements, such as diet, obesity, smoking, ethanol intake, and the effects of exercise.[8] Other variables include fed state, position while the sample is drawn, and the use and duration of venous occlusion; various anticoagulants and the storage and shipping conditions can alter lipoprotein measurements.[9]

Triglycerides have a well-described diurnal pattern and are affected by food ingestion; therefore, blood samples should be collected in the morning after a 10-hour fast. Excessive quantities of water should not be ingested prior to venous sampling. *The patient should be sitting quietly for approximately 15 minutes prior to blood drawing.* Positioning changes may result in alterations up to 12% in certain measured fractions. If multiple blood samples are required, then the lipid profile should be drawn first. Finger sticks are approximately 8.5% lower for all components measured.[9] EDTA is considered the standard anticoagulant for cholesterol measurement. Laboratories vary greatly on standards. If possible, the laboratory should meet CDC guidelines for accurate results.

Treatment

Diet, weight loss, and exercise are the most important components of first-level therapy. Books on cholesterol-lowering diets abound in most bookstores and allow the patient to choose a diet she (and her family) will best follow. The National Cholesterol Education Program recommends two step diets. The

Step-One diet limits dietary fats to 30% of daily intake with <10% saturated fats and 300 mg of cholesterol. After 3 months, lipids should be remeasured. If they are still elevated above recommended levels, then the Step-Two diet should be started. Saturated fats should be reduced to <7% and daily cholesterol intake reduced to 200 mg. Patients with poor family history for cardiovascular disease (history of premature coronary artery problems and strokes) should be tested and started on fat- and cholesterol-restricted diets in their twenties. After 3–6 months, if the LDL-cholesterol remains above 190 mg/dL without risk factors, or above 160 mg/dL with risk factors (listed in section introduction), then medical therapy should be initiated.

Estrogen replacement therapy should be first-line therapy in any postmenopausal patient. Bile acid binding resins were the only treatment option for years but were associated with abdominal bloating and gas, limiting their usefulness.[10] Representative drugs available are cholestyramine (4–16 grams daily) and colestipol (5–20 grams daily). Triglycerides are unaffected by these agents; however, they will lower LDL-cholesterol by 15–30% and raise HDL-cholesterol by 3–5%. An important side effect is potential binding of other medications.

Currently, there are two drugs commonly used: statins (lovastatin, pravastatin, simvastatin) and nicotinic acid. The usual dose of nicotinic acid is 500 mg three times a day, with a maximum dose of 1.0 gram four times a day. Nicotinic acid will usually lower LDL-cholesterol by 10–25% and triglycerides by 20–50% and elevate HDL-cholesterol by 15–35%. Facial flushing is a significant side effect but can be controlled with 325 mg of aspirin or 200 mg of ibuprofen 30 minutes prior to the first morning dose during the first 2 weeks of therapy.

In most patients a progressive dosing schedule for nicotinic may minimize side effects:

Week 1	125 mg bid
Week 2	250 mg bid
Weeks 3 and 4	500 mg bid
Week 5	1000 mg bid
Week 6	1500 mg bid

A long-acting formulation of nicotinic acid is available but is not FDA approved and is associated with a higher incidence of liver toxicity. The usual dosage is 1–2 grams once daily.

Lovastatin is a relatively new drug and the first introduced in its class. Initial dosing should be a single 20-mg dose at bedtime and may be increased to 40 mg twice a day. The metabolic consequences of lovastatin include a 20–40% reduction in LDL-cholesterol, 10–20% decrease in triglycerides, with a 5–10% increase in HDL-cholesterol. Lovastatin may cause muscle necrosis if combined with *nicotinic acid, erythromycin, cyclosporin, or fibric acid derivatives* (*clofibrate or gemfibrozil*). Creatinine kinase levels should be monitored. Patients on either medication should have a SGOT measurement after 6 and 12 weeks and then semiannually once therapeutic levels are reached.[11] In difficult to control cases, bile acid resins may be added to either medication. The goal of therapy is to lower LDL-cholesterol to less than 100 mg/dL.

Cholesterol measurements should be repeated after 1 month of therapy or 1 month after any alteration in therapy.

Patient involvement with dietary logs, cholesterol measurements, and so on may help in compliance.

Other Clinical Considerations. Pregnancy is associated with a decrease in total cholesterol in the first trimester. All fractions increase in the remaining trimesters.[12] The LDL and triglyceride concentrations are the lipoproteins most affected by pregnancy. Because of the limited studies in pregnancy and the radically altered metabolism, routine sampling is probably futile.

Certain disease states and medications impact on cholesterol measurements. As noted in the above section, diuretics and propranolol are noted to increase triglycerides and decrease HDL-cholesterol. Diuretics may also increase total cholesterol. Diabetics, especially those with poor control, may have very high levels of triglycerides and LDL-cholesterol and decreased HDL-cholesterol. This may explain why they are prone to cardiovascular diseases. Diabetics under "tight" control generally have improved lipoprotein levels.

Referral

Individuals with concurrent diseases such as coronary artery disease or difficult to control diabetes probably require more intensive therapy provided by an internist. If a patient fails to respond to diet and monotherapy with one of the above regimens, then referral is indicated. Failure of therapy would be indicated by continued levels of:

- Total cholesterol > 220 mg/dL
- LDL-cholesterol > 130 mg/dL

- HDL-cholesterol < 35 mg/dL
- Triglyceride levels > 250 mg/dL

Additionally, patients with initial levels of total cholesterol >300 mg/dL, or triglycerides of >400 mg/dL may have difficult to control congenital hyperlipidemias. Early referral may be the best course with these individuals.

▶ REFERENCES

1. Ladias JAA, Kwiterovich PO, Smith HH, et al. Apolipoprotein B-100 Hopkins (arginine$_{4019}$-tryptophan). *JAMA* 1989;262:1980–8.

2. Austin MA, Breslow JL, Hennekens CH, Buring JE, Willett WC, Krauss RM. Low-density lipoprotein subclass patterns and risk of myocardial infarction. *JAMA* 1988;260:1917–21.

3. Genest J Jr, McNamara JR, Ordovas JM, et al. Lipoprotein cholesterol, apolipoprotein A-I and B and lipoprotein (a) abnormalities in men with premature coronary artery disease. *J Am Coll Cardiol* 1992;19:792–802.

4. Soma MR, Osnago-Gadda I, Paoletti R, et al. The lowering of lipoprotein[a] induced by estrogen plus progesterone replacement therapy in postmenopausal women. *Arch Intern Med* 1993;153:1462–8.

5. Katan MB, Beynen AC. Characteristics of human hypo- and hyperresponders to dietary cholesterol. *Am J Epidemiol* 1987;125:387–99.

6. Ramsey LE, Yeo WW, Jackson PR. Dietary reduction of serum cholesterol concentration: time to think again. *Br Med J* 1991;303:953–7.

7. Naughton MJ, Luepker RV, Strickland D. The accuracy of portable cholesterol analyzers in public screening programs. *JAMA* 1990;263:1213–17.

8. Irwig L, Glaszious P, Wilson A, Macaskill P. Estimating an individual's true cholesterol level and response to intervention. *JAMA* 1991;266:1678–85.

9. Cooper GR, Myers GL, Smith SJ, Sampson EJ. Standardization of lipid, lipoprotein, and apolipoprotein measurements. *Clin Chem* 1988;34:B95–105.

10. Blum CB, Levy RI. Current therapy for hypercholesterolemia. *JAMA* 1989;261:3582–7.

11. Bradford RH, Shear CL, Chremos AN, et al. Expanded clinical evaluation of lovastatin (EXCEL) study results. *Arch Intern Med* 1991;151:43–9.

12. van Stiphout WAHJ, Hofman A, de Bruijn AM. Serum lipids in young women before, during, and after pregnancy. *Am J Epidemiol* 1987;126:922–8.

ENDOCRINE DISORDERS

Obstetricians and gynecologists have an intrinsic advantage over most physicians because the principles of endocrinology, such as feedback mechanisms, are fundamental to understanding conditions of the female reproductive tract. Chapter 8 deals with mostly type II diabetes or non–insulin-dependent diabetes mellitus (NIDDM). Most obstetricians and gynecologists are conversant in the care of the patient with type I or insulin-dependent diabetes mellitus (IDDM) based on their obstetric experience. The diagnosis and care of the patient with NIDDM is completely different, however, including the physiology of the disease. Most NIDDM patients do not manifest glucose intolerance until after age 40 and, hence, the condition is often diagnosed by internists.

Chapter 9 is concerned with thyroid function, especially in reference to changes that occur under hormonal influences. Thyroid disease is primarily a disease of women and may be difficult to diagnose because of the subtlety of early presentations. Hypothyroidism may easily be cared for by the primary care physician. Hyperthyroidism, depending on the endocrinologist's philosophy, is treated with different modalities such as radioiodine ablation or medications. Despite the approach, disorders should be diagnosed and medical care initiated prior to referral. Finally, issues of screening will be discussed; genetic issues are not well defined, but thyroid disease does tend to run in families. A high degree of suspicion is necessary to detect thyroid dysfunction, which may be elusive at times. Additionally, the management of thyroid nodules has changed in the past decade with the advent of fine needle aspiration and biopsy, which are discussed.

8

Diabetes Mellitus

Diabetes mellitus (DM) is a chronic disorder characterized by abnormal carbohydrate, protein, and fat metabolism from a deficiency or altered secretion or function of insulin. The disease is defined by fasting hyperglycemia or an abnormal oral glucose tolerance test (OGTT). The major complications of DM are related to vascular and metabolic complications. Only 50% of the estimated 14 million Americans with diabetes have been diagnosed. The importance of diabetic control is exemplified by the associated diseases:

- Blindness in adults (25 times more likely)
- Kidney disease (17 times more likely)
- Gangrene (5 times more likely)
- Heart disease and stroke (2 times more likely)

The primary focus of this section will be non-insulin-dependent diabetes rather then insulin-dependent because of the familiarity of obstetrical training with IDDM. NIDDM is a heterogeneous form of diabetes that commonly occurs in older age groups (>40 years), is more commonly familial than IDDM (concurrence in identical twins is about 90–95%, compared to 25–50% in IDDM). In contrast to an almost complete absence of insulin, NIDDM patients are unable to properly utilize insulin, resulting in insulin resistance. Characteristically, there is impaired glucose uptake in target tissues with a compensatory increase in insulin secretion and, hence, higher than normal circulating levels of insulin. Other associated conditions include hypertension and hyperlipidemia. Obesity is a covariable in 85% of affected patients. The etiology of NIDDM continues to be unknown but is speculated to be caused by defects in both insulin secretion and target tissue action.

The majority of NIDDM patients who were diagnosed at an early age in life and have exhausted insulin stores in the pancreas may eventually require injected insulin for control. These diabetics are called insulin-*requiring* diabetics as opposed to insulin-*dependent* diabetics (i.e., type I). When placed under severe stress, such as infection or surgery, they may develop diabetic ketoacidosis (DKA), but more often their mechanism of metabolic decompensation is a *hyperglycemic hyperosmolar nonketotic state* (HHNS).

Screening

Risk factors for DM are age greater than 40 years, adiposity, and family history of diabetes. Certain ethnic groups are at higher risk for the development of diabetes, including Pima Indians (35%), Native Americans (17%), Hispanics (12%), and African–Americans (5%). The background rate for the general population is ≤2.5%. Life-style may be the most important variable for type II diabetes (non-insulin-dependent diabetes mellitus or NIDDM).

Disease classification is important in understanding the

metabolic and clinical differences in the diseases and will help in management decisions.

Major Classification

Type I: Insulin-dependent diabetes mellitus (IDDM)

Type II: Non-insulin-dependent diabetes mellitus (NIDDM) (subgroups of obese or nonobese)

Other Types of Diabetes

Pancreatic disease

Endocrinopathies (Cushing's syndrome, acromegaly, pheochromocytoma, hyperaldosteronism)

Drug-induced

Impaired glucose tolerance (IGT) (subgroups of obese or nonobese)

Different risk factors exist between type I and type II diabetes mellitus. Prevalence of IDDM is increased in siblings/parents, and highest in identical twins (25–50%). Most obstetricians and gynecologists have experience in the management of IDDM patients in pregnancy. Most patients present in childhood and adolescence and rarely in adulthood. NIDDM patients usually present after age 40. Risk factors for NIDDM are ethnicity, obesity, strong family history of DM, sedentary life-style, impaired glucose tolerance, upper body adiposity, history of gestational diabetes, and hyperinsulinemia. These risk factors strongly influence the development of NIDDM in susceptible individuals.

Risk factors that should alert the clinician that screening is necessary include:

- Persons with classic signs and symptoms of diabetes (i.e., polyuria, polydipsia, polyphagia, and loss of weight)
- Obesity
- Strong family history of diabetes
- Ethnic groups at high risk (Pima Indians, Native Americans, African–Americans, Hispanics)
- Morbid obstetrical history (defined as a history of macrosomia, shoulder dystocia)
- History of recurring skin, genital, or urinary tract infections, especially *Monilia*

The role of the oral glucose tolerance test is to assist in borderline cases. However, there can be as many as 10% false positives (guidelines met, but the disease is not clinically evident). The patient with borderline values should be started on life-style adjustments rather than medications.

Treatment

The following guidelines are for the general care of any class of diabetics and have long-term implications. (See Figure 8-1.)

- Establish diagnosis of diabetes mellitus (DM) and classify as outlined above.
- Do not perform OGTT if diagnosis of DM is already established.
- Initiate diabetes education classes (to learn signs and symptoms of loss of glycemic control, complications, blood glucose monitoring, diabetic medications, sick days, etc.).

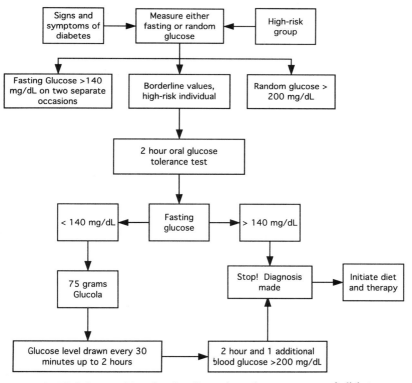

FIGURE 8-1. Algorithm for the diagnosis and management of diabetes mellitus.

- Place patient on ADA diet with appropriate caloric, sodium, and lipid restrictions.
- Establish cardiac risk factors such as tobacco use and hypertension.

- Establish baseline status of kidney function (serum creatinine, 24-hour urine albumin). Evaluate for presence of neuropathy (e.g., 1+ albumin on dipstick, presence of difficult to control hypertension, serum creatinine > 1.5 mg/dL and refer to neurologist if symptomatic.
- Establish extent of fundoscopic lesion or refer to ophthalmologist.
- Check feet and toenails at each visit.
- Use finger-stick blood glucose for daily diabetic control and check urine for ketones (but do not use first morning void).
- Follow chronic glycemic control by HgA_{1c} every 2–3 months (q 6 months in elderly) in the office.

Initial general health evaluation should consist of a complete history and physical examination and the following laboratory tests: CBC with differential, chemistry profile, lipid profile, urinalysis, thyroid function tests, and EKG (if indicated, baseline at age 40 or older).

Treatment of NIDDM

Diet continues to be the most important component of management and unfortunately is the hardest to achieve. The approach to overweight diabetics consists of three major strategies: weight loss, low-fat diet ($\leq$30% of calories from fat), and physical exercise. Obese patients should be advised to reduce to their ideal body weight. Advantages of weight reduction are improved lipid levels (lower triglycerides, total cholesterol, and LDL-cholesterol with increased HDL-cholesterol) and improved glucose control secondary to increased insulin sensitivity and decreased insulin resistance. Even a 10-pound weight loss will improve glucose and lipid measurements. Physical exercise helps with weight loss and improves insulin sensitivity and lipid levels especially for those at high risk for cardiovascular and microvascular diseases. General guidelines for management are the following:

- Place patient on ADA reducing diet (50% carbohydrates, 30% fat, 20% protein, high fiber) with three meals a day to achieve and maintain ideal body weight or to reduce weight by 5–15% in 3 months (if >130% above ideal body weight).

- Encourage risk factor modification (smoking, sedentary life-style, fat intake, etc.).

- After initiating diet, check fasting blood glucose (FBG) by finger stick daily for 2 months. If FBG gradually declines during this period, no other therapy is needed. If FBG does not decline or increases, consider use of oral hypo-glycemic agents (OHAs) if
  (1) patient has had diabetes for less than 10 years;
  (2) patient does not have severe hepatic or renal disease; and
  (3) patient is not allergic to sulfonylurea.

- Patients with FBG levels ≥250 mg/dL (after adequate dietary restriction) are not suitable candidates for OHA.

- While on OHAs, patients should have their FBG and two postprandial levels checked every 2 months in the office (in conjunction with daily home glucose monitoring [HGM]). If postprandial glucose < 200 mg/dL, diet alone is all that is necessary along with follow-up blood glucose tests every 1–2 months. If FBG levels are consistently >200 mg/dL, insulin therapy should be started.

- Insulin dosage should be calculated on *actual* body weight (0.5–1.0 Unit per kg body weight).

- If total insulin requirement is less than 30 U/day, consider giving the entire dose as NPH or Lente before a major meal. Goals for glucose control are: FBG < 140, 2 hr PP < 200, and no blood sugar < 60 mg/dL.

- If a single insulin injection is inadequate, insulin may be given as a mixture of regular/NPH (50:50) in split doses, $\frac{1}{2}$ hour before breakfast and $\frac{1}{2}$ hour before supper.

- Very obese NIDDM patients may require more insulin/kg body weight and a greater percentage of total insulin as regular insulin.

- Consider multiple regular insulin injections before each meal with bedtime NPH or Lente insulin.

Oral Hypoglycemic Agents—Sulfonylureas. Oral hypoglycemic agents (OHAs) are recommended for many NIDDM patients. First and second generation sulfonylureas are currently the only agents approved by the FDA. Other OHAs may be available in the near future with a different mechanism of action from sulfonylureas. Currently available formulations are listed in Table 8-1.

The mode of action of sulfonylureas results from two different mechanisms. They enhance insulin secretion from the pancreas and also provide an extrapancreatic effect. The lowest possible dose should be initiated and maintained. *OHAs have little effect on patients whose endogenous insulin secretion (as measured by C-peptide) is absent or the FBG on adequate diabetic diet is greater than 250 mg/dL.* The annual failure rate

▶ **TABLE 8-1   Formulations of Available Sulfonylureas**

OHA	Tradename	Daily Dose	Duration of Action (in hours)
Tolbutamide	Orinase	750 mg–3.0 g, divided doses	6–12
Tolazamide	Tolinase	200–1000 mg, divided doses	12–24
Acetohexamide	Dymelor	250–1500 mg, single dose	12–24
Chlorpropamide	Diabinese	100–500 mg, single dose	Up to 60
Glyburide	Micronase, DiaBeta	2.5–20 mg, variable dose	10–24
Glipizide	Glucotrol	2.5–40 mg, variable dose	3–8

of glucose control with oral agents is 3–5%. Frequent evaluation to monitor control (every 2 months) is important.

Insulin Therapy in NIDDM. A combination of an evening dose of insulin (NPH or combined NPH + regular) at supper or bedtime, followed by a morning dose of OHA may be effective in the control of hyperglycemia. This method is controversial and may be better handled by referral. The newly available fixed combinations of NPH and regular insulin (70/30; 50/50) may be reasonable to use in this group of patients.

Assessment of Glycemic Control. The only acceptable method for assessment of glycemic control is blood glucose determination. Many studies have confirmed the absence of correlation between blood glucose and urine glucose. Techniques using strips and meters are available that are adequate for glucose determination. The accuracy of such machines has been well documented, but it is important to remember results are *whole blood determinations, not serum.* Strips for blood glucose readings use color for sugar levels and require some interpretation, which may be difficult for the elderly or the colorblind. Glucometers with memory storage have made home glucose monitoring more acceptable to patients and health care providers. Urine test tapes for ketones remain useful and quick in assessing ketosis. Patients should check their urine for ketones if their sugar levels are elevated, and/or seek medical advice when their blood glucose levels remain above 300 mg/dL. Infection remains the most common cause for lack of glycemic control in the compliant patient.

Glycohemoglobin. Patients who are unreliable or unable to perform HGM are difficult to manage. Additionally, diabetics are notorious for not reporting accurate glucose control. In conditions where chronic glycemic assessments are desirable, glycohemoglobin is assayed. Glycohemoglobin is a product of a ketoamine reaction between glucose in the blood and N-terminal amino acids of the beta chains of hemoglobin and consist of hemoglobin A_{1a}, A_{1b}, and A_{1c}. The glycohemogloblin level generally reflects the glycemic state over the previous 12 weeks (the approximate half-life of a red cell). The normal level of HbA_{1c} is between 4% and 6% (depending on the laboratory method used). Most diabetologists consider values up to 7% as excellent control, while values above 10% are considered poor control. Falsely decreased levels of glycosylated hemoglobin are found in patients with severe anemia or shortened red blood cell half-life, as in hemolytic anemias or hemoglobinopathies.

Referral

Individual patients who do not respond to diet and OHAs may best be referred due to the complexity of the problem. Usually these patients are obese and hypertensive, with other diseases, and are better served by an internist. Patients with vascular disease or other medical disorders should also be referred. Unreliable patients, the bane of any practitioner's practice, should be referred to a diabetologist, if reasonable. If an insulin-resistant stage is reached (defined as >200 U insulin/day), then referral to a diabetologist is indicated.

9

Thyroid Disease

    Thyroid disorders are more common in women than men by a ratio of approximately 10:1. There is a familial tendency; however, the exact pattern of inheritance has not been determined. Thyroid dysfunction may affect up to 2–3% of the population and is especially prevalent in the elderly. The diagnosis of thyroid disease can be difficult because it has many elusive presentations. Several states common to reproductive-age women, such as pregnancy and the use of exogenous hormones, may obscure the actual disease or lead to a false diagnosis. With the advent of sensitive thyroid-stimulating hormone (TSH) assays, hormonal alterations have become less important in screening. Altered hormonal states must be considered in the interpretation of thyroxine levels, however. Consequently, the knowledge of thyroid physiology in women is vital for obstetricians and gynecologists. Because of the multitude of abbreviations, Table 9-1 should be reviewed before proceeding with the discussion.

► CLINICAL PHYSIOLOGY

Thyroid hormones become active in target tissues by binding in nuclear receptors. Thyroxine (T_4), the main product of the

▶ TABLE 9-1   Common Abbreviations in Thyroid Physiology

TRH: Thyroid-releasing hormone. Hypothalamic regulatory hormone.

TSH: Thyroid-stimulating hormone. Pituitary regulatory hormone, stimulated by TRH and with negative feedback by peripheral hormones.

T_3: Triiodothyronine. Active thryoid hormone, primarily by peripheral conversion of thyroxine (T_4).

T_4: Thyroxine: Primary hormone released from thyroid gland, requires peripheral conversion to T_3 to become activated. Commonly given for replacement therapy.

TBG: Thyroxin-binding globulin. Synthesized in the liver and specific carrier protein for thyroxine. Affected by hormones such as estrogen and testosterone.

TSI: Thyroid-stimulating immunoglobulin. IgG antibody that stimulates pituitary to produce inappropriate high levels of TSH. May pass placenta, causing neonatal hyperthyroidism.

---

thyroid gland, provides a stable reservoir for extrathyroidal conversion to triiodothyronine (T_3). The more biologically active of the two hormones, T_3 also has a higher affinity for the nuclear receptor. Pituitary TSH regulates hormone production and thyroid growth. It is regulated by hypothalamic thyrotropin-releasing hormone (TRH) using a classic negative feedback mechanism. Thyroid-stimulating immunoglobulin (TSI), formerly referred to as long-acting thyroid stimulator (LATS), binds to the TSH receptor and is the cause of hyperthyroid Graves' disease.

Over 99% of circulating T_4 and T_3 is bound by plasma proteins, predominantly thyroxinbinding globulin (TBG). The quantity of free levels of thyroid hormone in circulating serum proteins remains constant despite physiologic or pharmacologic alterations. Changes in total serum protein levels have no effect on the patient's clinical status. Estrogen, regardless of its source, increases TBG plasma concentration by decreasing hepatic clearance. Androgens, especially testosterone, and corticosteroids have the opposite effect by increasing TBG clearance. Elevated thyroid hormone concentrations may be the result of increased protein binding from altered albumin and estrogen states and decreased peripheral conversion of T_4 and T_3.

Thyroid function test results may be misleading in women taking certain drugs (i.e., propranolol and amiodarone) or who have systemic illnesses (i.e., malignancy, sepsis, multiple organ failure, and acute renal failure). Hyperemesis gravidarum may cause very low TSH and T_4 levels. Transitions from puberty to menopause do not alter free thyroid hormone concentrations.

Screening

The patient's neck should be palpated during routine physical examinations. Patients who are exposed to radiation, even low doses, are at increased risk of thyroid carcinoma. Because of the high number of asymptomatic nodules detected with ultrasound—up to 30% in some series—it should not be utilized for routine screening.[1]

With the exception of neonates, laboratory testing of asymptomatic patients has not been found to be cost effective.[2] Early treatment of thyroid disease has not been shown to modify the course of the disease. Elderly patients may have disease without symptoms, however, which compounds the problem. Detection may be helpful in the elderly where psychiatric and some medical disorders have been attributed to disturbances other than thyroid disease.

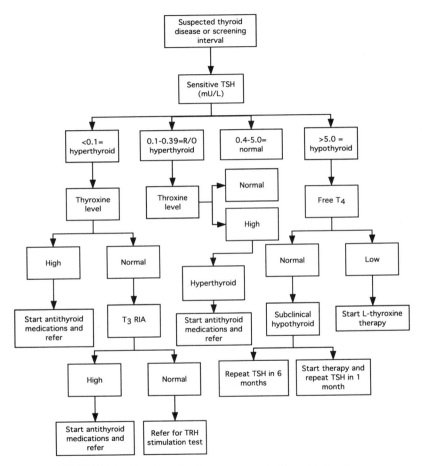

FIGURE 9-1. Algorithm for the management of thyroid disorders.

Because thyroid disease is prevalent in some families, periodic screening may be justified. Unfortunately, there are no set guidelines or recommendations for periodic screening.[3] It is probably reasonable to screen patients with familial tendencies, autoimmune diseases, and unfavorable lipid profiles every 3 years between the ages of 19 and 39 years and every 2 years afterward. After age 40, screening may be performed every 5 years in all patients. Women under 65 should be considered for screening biannually, especially if psychiatric disease is present.[4] Currently, there are no guidelines for screening.

Because of the absence of hormonal influence in sensitive TSH assays, this test should be used instead of thyroxine assays for screening. Fortunately, the ultrasensitive TSH assay has eliminated the problem of TBG binding alterations caused by hormonal changes.[3] An algorithm for interpretation and management of abnormal TSH levels and goiters is shown in Figure 9-1.

Diagnosis

Manifestations of hypothyroidism include fatigue, lethargy, cold intolerance, nightmares, dry skin, hair loss, constipation, myalgia, carpal tunnel syndrome, and weight gain, which is usually less than 5–10 kg. Menstrual dysfunction is common; menorrhagia is the most frequent abnormality, and amenorrhea can occur. Anovulatory women who have normal thyroid function do not benefit from thyroid replacement therapy. Common neuropsychiatric symptoms include depression, irritability, impaired memory, and, in the elderly, dementia. Individuals with amenorrhea, galactorrhea, and hyperprolactinemia should undergo TSH testing to distinguish primary hypothyroidism from a prolactin-secreting pituitary adenoma.

Patients with hyperthyroidism experience fatigue, diarrhea, heat intolerance, palpitations, dyspnea, nervousness, and weight loss. Paradoxically, young patients may have weight gain due to increased appetite. Tachycardia, lid lag, tremor, proximal muscle weakness, and warm moist skin are often present. Ophthalmologic changes include lid retraction, periorbital edema, and proptosis, but these changes occur in less than one-third of women with hyperthyroidism. In the elderly, symptoms may be more subtle and include unexplained weight loss, atrial fibrillation, or new-onset angina pectoris. Most thyrotoxic patients have regular menses with lighter flow; however, anovulatory menses and associated infertility are common. Goiter is common in younger women but may be absent in the elderly. Toxic nodular goiter is associated with non-homogeneous glandular enlargement. Subacute thyroiditis is associated with a tender, hard, and enlarged gland.

Treatment

Hypothyroidism. The treatment of choice for hypothyroidism is L-thyroxine (T_4). The mode of action of T_4 is identical to that of endogenous thyroid—conversion to T_3 in peripheral tissues. A parenteral formulation is available but rarely necessary, because of the long half-life (7 days) of oral preparations. Aluminum hydroxide (common in antacids), cholestyramine, ferrous sulfate, or sucralfate can either bind or chelate oral preparations and interfere with absorption. Additionally, dosage may require adjustment with antiepileptic drugs. The T_4 dose requirement is weight related (approximately 1.6 μg/kg) and decreases in the elderly. Formulations are commonly available in 0.025 mg increments. The normal daily dose is 0.1– 0.15 mg, but the final dosage should be adjusted to maintain the serum TSH within the normal range. In pregnant women, the T_4 dose requirement is increased by 25–100%, but the final dosage should be adjusted by monitoring the serum TSH. Thyroid status should be assessed between 8 and 12 weeks and again between 20 and 24 weeks. The prepregnancy dosage can be resumed immediately postpartum.

Thyroid replacement should be monitored approximately 3 weeks after initiation of therapy or after medication adjustments. Even a mild increase of T_4 above normal levels has been associated with cortical bone loss and osteoporosis. A low initial T_4 dose (0.0125–0.025 mg/day) should be initiated in patients with known or suspected coronary artery disease because rapid replacement may worsen angina and induce myocardial infarction.

Hyperthyroidism. Unless the patient is pregnant, referral for therapy should be considered after the initial diagnosis and initiation of medication. The mainstay of therapy for hyperthyroidism is antithyroid medication, either propylthiouracil (PTU 50–300 mg every 6–8 hours) or methimazole (Tapazole® 10–30 mg/day). Both antithyroid drugs block thyroid hormone biosynthesis. Additionally, PTU partially inhibits extrathyroidal T_4-to-T_3 conversion, but methimazole has a longer half-life and can be administered in a single daily dose.

Antithyroid medications have infrequent (5%) minor side effects, which include fever, rash, and arthralgias. Major drug toxicity is rare (<1%); when toxicity occurs it causes hepatitis, vasculitis, and agranulocytosis. Agranulocytosis usually presents as strep throat. Any patient who complains of orophagia should be evaluated and treated with antibiotics.

Lifelong follow-up is warranted in patients who opt for medical therapy due to the high relapse rate. Most relapses occur in the postpartum period. The euthyroid state is typically restored within 3–10 weeks. Approximately 50% of individuals treated with medication alone will have a recurrence and possible thyroid storm (fever, tachycardia, abdominal pain). Treatment is continued for 6–24 months, unless total ablation by radioiodine or surgery is performed. Thyroid ablation by radioiodine results in permanent hypothyroidism. Surgery is expensive and invasive, and it may result in inadvertent parathyroid removal, which commits the patient to lifelong calcium therapy.

Ablation therapy with iodine-131 provides a permanent cure of hyperthyroidism in 70–80% of patients. The principal drawback to radioactive iodine therapy is the high rate of postablative hypothyroidism. Most medical endocrinologists assume that hypothyroidism will develop and recommend that patients receive thyroid replacement therapy for the remainder of their lifetime. The estimated ovarian exposure to radiation is minimal (1–2 rads), essentially the same as widely employed diagnostic procedures (e.g., barium enema with fluoroscopy and hysterosalpingography).

Beta-adrenergic blocking drugs are useful adjunctive therapy to control sympathomimetic symptoms in patients with hyperthyroidism. These medications offer the additional benefit of blocking peripheral conversion of T_4 to T_3. If thyroid storm occurs, PTU, beta-blocking agents, glucocorticoids, and high-dose iodine preparations (supersaturated potassium iodide [SSKI], or intravenous sodium iodide) should be administered. Admission to an intensive care facility is advisable, but therapy should be initiated in the emergency department prior to transport.

Thyroid Nodules. Thyroid nodules are common and may be found during physical examination in up to 5% of patients.

Most nodules are asymptomatic when discovered and are usually benign; however, malignancy and hyperthyroidism must be excluded. Previous radiation exposure, even to low doses during childhood, is associated with a higher risk of malignancy.[5] Virtually all nodules require evaluation. In the past decade this has been accomplished by fine needle aspiration and biopsy (FNAB), as shown in Figure 9-2. Prior to performing FNAB, thyroid function should be tested. If hypothyroidism or hyperthyroidism is detected, appropriate therapy should be initiated, which may eliminate the nodule. Biopsy should be performed on nodules that persist after therapy. Most nodules are "cold" on scanning or imaging; therefore, it is more cost effective to proceed directly to tissue sampling. Fine needle biopsy is successful in most cases, and only in 5% of cases is surgical biopsy required. Only 20% of surgical biopsies of an "indeterminate aspiration" are found to be malignant.

Approximately 75% of malignancies are papillary thyroid carcinoma. Cure rates are >90%, even in the presence of cervical lymph node metastases, when patients are less than 50 years of age and the primary tumor is less than 4 cm at presentation. Anaplastic tumors in the elderly have a poor prognosis and usually progress rapidly despite therapy. Radioiodine therapy or surgical ablation are the most common methods of therapy. Regardless of the form of treatment used, lifetime thyroxine suppression therapy should be administered.

In a pregnant woman with a thyroid nodule, FNAB should be performed followed by thyroxine suppression therapy. If malignancy is strongly suspected, surgical exploration may be performed in the second trimester. If the nodule is not suspicious, FNAB may be delayed until after delivery. With papillary carcinoma, either immediate surgery or thyroxine suppression (until surgery can be performed during the postpartum

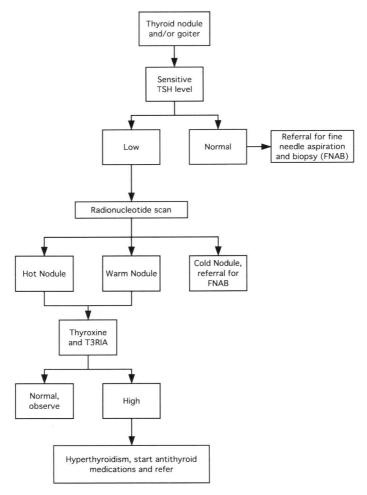

FIGURE 9-2. Algorithm for the management of a thyroid nodule.

period) is acceptable. When more aggressive histology is found, surgery is indicated.

Referral

In cases of simple hypothyroidism, the gynecologist should be the primary care physician. In cases of hyperthyroidism, referral should be considered because of the expertise and equipment needed to use medications such as cytomel and radioiodine. After ablation, however, monitoring thyroid replacement therapy is well within the expertise of the gynecologist. Thyroid nodules should be referred for FNAB in most cases. Additionally, neck exploration (which is a dying art) may best be performed by an otolaryngologist.

▶ REFERENCES

1. Ezzat S, Sarti DA, Cain DR, Braunstein GD. Thyroid incidentalomas. *Arch Intern Med* 1994;154:1838–40.

2. Report of the United States Preventative Services Task Force. *Screening for thyroid disease*. Baltimore: William & Wilkins, 1991;105–10.

3. Surks MI, Chopra IJ, Marisash CN, Nicoloff JT, Solomon DH. American Thyroid Association guidelines for use of laboratory tests in thyroid disorders. *JAMA* 1990;263:1529–32.

4. Helfand M, Crapo LM. Screening for thyroid disease. *Ann Intern Med* 1990;112:840–9.

5. Shimaoka K, Bakri K, Sciascia M, et al. Thyroid screening program: follow-up evaluation. *N Y State J Med* 1982;82:1184–7.

NONGYNECOLOGIC CANCER

Primary care physicians should be aware of two diseases that continue to cause significant morbidity and mortality in women: breast and colorectal cancers. Both of these cancers have a much better prognosis when they are diagnosed in early stages. Screening issues for both diseases have been the subject of great debate: when to begin mammography and the role of fecal occult blood testing. Chapter 10 deals with the diagnosis of breast cancer and current recommendations for screening. Mammography screening may have a major impact on the stage of disease at the time of diagnosis and long-term mortality. Therapeutic options have changed in the past decade for early disease, with less aggressive surgical therapies used with equal success to more extensive procedures. The emergence of lumpectomy and radiation therapy, avoiding disfiguring surgery, is a welcome change from the old radical mastectomy for all patients.

Colorectal cancer remains a major cause of death for men and women. Chapter 11 reviews the major risk factors and presents a screening algorithm. Screening issues remain controversial, and the role of fecal occult blood testing has not been resolved. Screening flexible sigmoidoscopy may become a major tool in early identification of colon cancer, especially if its use becomes widespread. As practices regarding reimbursement for endoscopy procedures change, the cost/benefit ratio may promote more widespread flexible sigmoidoscopy screening. It is relatively easy to learn to perform screening sigmoidoscopy, and the procedure may become a valuable addition to the practice of obstetrics and gynecology.

Breast Disorders

Breast cancer is the most common invasive cancer that occurs in women and the malignancy most often encountered in women by primary care physicians. It represents 32% of the cancers in women and causes 18% of the deaths from cancer. The National Cancer Institute estimates that one in nine women has a lifetime risk for the development of breast cancer. It is estimated that one in four women in the United States will require medical care for breast problems, most of which are benign. Symptoms of breast disease often motivate women to consult their physicians. Unfortunately, failure to diagnose breast cancer is a major cause of litigation involving obstetrician–gynecologists in the United States.

The obstetrician–gynecologist who is a primary care provider for women should offer patients regular clinical breast examinations (CBEs), instruction on breast self-examination (BSE), screening mammography, and the evaluation of signs and symptoms of breast disease. The diagnosis of breast disease and the treatment of benign breast conditions may be performed easily in the office setting.

Screening

Mammography is currently the only effective screening method for detecting nonpalpable breast cancers, which, when

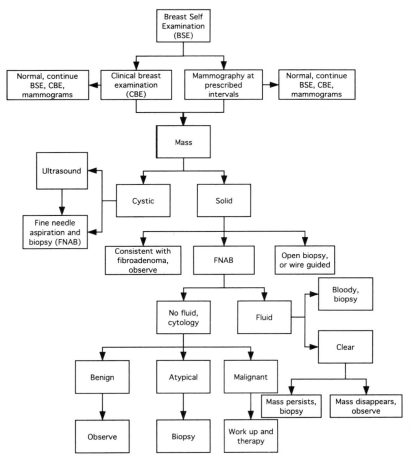

FIGURE 10-1. Algorithm for the management of breast disease.

treated, have an excellent prognosis. Both BSE and CBE by the practitioner are still important for early detection; however, BSE has not been shown as effective as once thought.[1] Screening for breast cancer should include CBE because of high false-negative rates for mammography. Multiple studies have shown that the false-negative rate for mammography may be as high as 30% in patients under 40 years of age to 10% in patients over 60 years of age.[2] Although BSE has not shown improvement in the overall survival of treated breast cancer patients, there may be some value to the procedure.[3] Regular BSE promotes women's awareness of anatomical variations and encourages them to consult their physicians about breast changes, signs, and symptoms (Figure 10-1).

Clinical Breast Examination. A systematic method should be used to most effectively perform the CBE. A visual examination should be performed with the patient sitting with her hands placed on her hips and her shoulders pulled back. Another helpful maneuver is to push the palms together to flex the pectoralis major muscle. Breast symmetry and contour should be noted, in addition to any scars or skin changes. If a breast mass is palpated, the patient should be examined in both the supine and upright positions. Any adenopathy of the axilla or supraclavicular area should be noted. Precise recording of the performance of the CBE and any clinically significant findings is essential. Because of the effect of the menstrual cycle on masses, if any indistinct lesion is palpated, especially in the luteal phase, the examination should be repeated after the next menstrual period.

Breast Self-Examination. Guidelines from the American College of Obstetricians and Gynecologists (ACOG) recommend that women should be instructed in BSE beginning at age 18. The patient should demonstrate her interpretation of BSE after instruction, and educational material should be provided. Breast self-examination is best performed a few days after the cessation of menstruation or, if the woman is not menstruating, monthly on the same calendar day. The importance of performing BSE should be reinforced during each annual gynecologic visit.

Mammography. Current ACOG guidelines recommend mammography screening to be initiated at age 40 and performed every 1–2 years until age 50. After age 50, mammography should be performed annually. A patient who has a family history of breast cancer in a first-degree relative (mother or sister) should begin annual screening mammography 10 years earlier than the age of the first-degree relative when cancer was diagnosed. Despite this recommendation, there are no studies proving the efficacy of this protocol.[4]

The cost effectiveness of screening mammography for women younger than age 50 is a consideration. Many physicians recommend biannual screening mammography beginning at age 40 although statistically significant data are not available (probably because of inadequate statistical power) to validate the effectiveness of screening mammography for women under age 50. Thus far, studies do not support the need for mammography in women under age 50.[5]

The physician who ordered the mammography examination should receive a report of the results, which should be communicated to the patient. Abnormalities should be discussed with the radiologist and, if possible, reviewed. It is helpful to have the patient obtain a copy of a previous mammogram for comparison. Because of the risk of false-positive results,[6] any suspicious palpable mass should be biopsied.

History

Numerous epidemiologic factors—high socioeconomic level, high dietary fat intake, early age of menarche, late age of menopause, and obesity—have been linked to a risk for breast cancer, but the association is weak. The strongest risk factor for breast cancer is a woman's advancing age. Maintaining body weight within the normal range for age and height and limiting alcohol intake to moderate levels have shown in some studies to slightly decrease breast cancer relative risk, but the data are conflicting. Reproductive risk factors—nulliparity, older age at first birth, early menarche, late menopause, preventive effect of lactation, and use of hormone replacement therapy—are important in assessing risk.

A personal history of breast cancer and breast cancer in a first-degree relative significantly increases a woman's relative risk of breast cancer. These patients have familial breast cancer (FBC), in contrast to hereditary breast cancer (HBC). Hereditary breast cancer syndromes have been described in some families with an autosomal dominant inheritance with high penetrance.[7] Patients with genital cancers may also be at higher risk for breast cancer and screening should be initiated even at younger ages.

With the exception of breast cancer in a first-degree relative, history is rarely helpful in diagnosing breast cancer. Identified risk factors do not provide insight into the cause or control of the disease, and they do not apply to approximately 80% of women with breast cancer.

Diagnosis

The diagnostic triad of CBE, mammography, and fine needle aspiration (FNA) will usually yield a definitive diagnosis of most palpable breast neoplasms.[8] Ultrasound can be useful to determine if a questionable area is cystic and thus may be observed without biopsy; it is not a primary diagnostic tool, however. In most cases, FNA can be used to establish a specific cytologic diagnosis if an adequate cell sample is obtained. Needle core biopsy may be performed, but it is more invasive, has more complications (such as bleeding), and requires a local anesthetic and often a suture for skin closure. If a diagnosis cannot be confirmed with these procedures, open surgical biopsy must be performed. Localizing breast masses using a wire guided by mammography may be useful in diagnosing smaller masses.

Fibroadenomas commonly occur in the early reproductive years, cysts in the middle and late reproductive years, and cancers in the peri- and postmenopausal years. However, age ranges overlap and should never be used as diagnostic criteria. A persistent, dominant breast mass must be diagnosed.

Palpable cysts may readily be diagnosed and treated by FNA.[9] After aspiration of cyst fluid, the area should be palpated or repeat mammography should be performed to establish that there is no residual or underlying mass. The breast should be reexamined within 3 months to assure that the cyst has not recurred. A repeat FNA may be performed, but recurrence of cyst fluid suggests a neoplastic etiology and biopsy or removal may be the best course. Cytologic assessment of cyst fluid and nipple discharge is rarely diagnostic, even in the presence of bloody fluid. In many cases, benign cells in the cyst fluid are interpreted as "atypical" and require further diagnostic procedures (needle core or open biopsy) to rule out neoplasia.

Fibroadenomas are the most common benign neoplasms of the breast and have a unique appearance on mammography. In most patients, these tumors appear at a young age, but age should not be a diagnostic criterion. A definitive cytologic diagnosis of a palpable fibroadenoma usually can be established with FNA. Once a fibroadenoma is diagnosed, the condition should be monitored. There is no associated premalignant potential; however, the patient may elect to have the fibroadenoma removed. This is usually performed as outpatient surgery under local anesthesia.

As many as 75% of women may elicit some nipple discharge with persistent squeezing. Pathologic nipple discharge from an intrinsic lesion is spontaneous, usually unilateral, and emitted from a single duct opening on the nipple. Ductography (galactography) is effective in demonstrating intraductal lesions causing nipple discharge but unreliable in differentiating benign intraductal papillomas from papillary cancers. Therefore, all intraductal lesions that produce a nipple discharge should be completely excised. Mammary duct ectasia (periductal mastitis), commonly found in the perimenopausal years, produces a dark discharge from multiple nipple duct openings and usually is self-limited. Surgical treatment is usually necessary if it is persistent.

Treatment

Most obstetricians and gynecologists are involved in the diagnosis of breast masses and not treatment of cancer. After establishing the absence of breast cancer, either by the diagnostic triad or by histology, certain benign breast diseases are amenable to treatment in the office setting.

Controversy exists over whether caffeine contributes to mastalgia with fibrocystic disease; however, limitation of caffeine may be beneficial in some patients. Mastalgia is a common breast complaint, particularly in young women. Because of the widespread focus on breast cancer, many of these patients fear they have a malignancy. After evaluation by the diagnostic triad, many women with a chief complaint of mastalgia and without an associated dominant mass can be appropriately managed by reassurance. A trial of mechanical (brassier changes), dietary, and analgesic interventions should be initiated. If conservative measures are unsuccessful, treatment with low-dose birth control pills may be helpful. Danazol is the only pharmacologic treatment approved for mastalgia, but in most cases the side effects (masculinization) are unacceptable to patients.

Referral

In many cases, referral will be dictated by the level of comfort and training the physician has in treating breast disease. In many cases, most gynecologists will perform cyst aspiration but not FNA and open biopsy. Once cancer is diagnosed, referral to a surgeon and oncologist is customary.

► REFERENCES

1. O'Malley MS, Fletcher SW. US Preventative Services Task Force. Screening for breast cancer with breast self-examination: a critical review. *JAMA* 1987;257:2196–203.

2. Coveney EC, Geraghty JG, O'Laoide R, Hourihane JB, O'Higgins NJ. Reasons underlying negative mammography in patients with palpable breast cancer. *Clin Radiol* 1994;49:2123–5.

3. O'Malley MS, Fletcher SW. Screening for breast cancer with breast self examination. *JAMA* 1987;257:2197–293.

4. Vogel VG. Screening younger women at risk for breast cancer. *Monogr Natl Cancer Inst* 1994;16:55–60.

5. Miller AB, Baines CL, To T, et al. Canadian national breast screening study: 1. Breast cancer and death rates among women aged 40 to 49 years. *Can Med Assoc J* 1992;147:1459–76.

6. Svane G, Potchen EJ, Siena A, et al. How to interpret a mammogram. In: *Screening mammography–breast cancer diagnosis in asymptomatic women.* St. Louis: Mosby, 1993;148–201.

7. Marcus JN, Watson P, Page DL, Lynch HT. Pathology and heredity of breast cancer in younger women. *Monogr Natl Cancer Inst* 1994;16:23–34.

8. Hindle WH. Breast masses: in-office evaluation with diagnostic triad. *Postgrad Med* 1990;88:85–94.

9. Costa MJ, Tadros T, Hilton G, Birdsong G. Breast fine needle aspiration cytology. Utility as a screening tool for clinically palpable lesions. *Acta Cytol* 1993;37(4):461–71.

CHAPTER 11

Colorectal Cancer

Colorectal cancer is the second most common cancer in the United States. An estimated 160,000 new cases occur each year, usually in individuals over age 50, with an annual mortality rate of 60,000. The sites of origin have changed from being predominantly in the rectum to being equally distributed between the rectum and the proximal descending colon. Genetic predisposition (a deletion on chromosome 5)[1] is reported to be associated with the colorectal cancer and is currently being actively investigated. Large-bowel cancers may be related to environmental factors. Risk factors include high socioeconomic level in urban areas, high level of dietary fat and meat protein intake, hypercholesterolemia, and coronary artery disease.[2] In contrast, Seventh Day Adventists, who are vegetarians, have a lower incidence of colorectal cancer.

Two theories (transit time and bacterial content) have been presented to clarify the relationship between dietary influences and the occurrence of colorectal carcinoma. Stools of individuals in areas with a high prevalence of colorectal cancer have been cultured and found to be high in anaerobic flora. These microorganisms convert bile salts to carcinogens. High-fiber diets, which are common in Africa, are associated with a reduced occurrence of bowel cancers. High-fiber diets are thought to increase stool transit time, limiting bowel wall con-

143

tact with potential carcinogens in fecal material. Because there are multiple other cultural considerations, these theories continue to be speculative. The symptoms of bowel cancer are nonspecific and do not correlate with either the stage of disease or prognosis. Therefore, screening becomes an important issue in identifying and curing early disease.

History

Colorectal carcinomas have been associated with multiple syndromes and high-risk groups[3]:

- Gardner's syndrome (small and large intestine)
- Familial colonic polyposis (large intestine)
- Turcot's syndrome (large intestine)
- Nonpolyposis syndrome (large intestine)
- Cancer family syndrome (large intestine, ovary, endometrial)
- Ulcerative colitis (large intestine)
- Family history of cancers:
    a) Gynecologic—cervix, endometrial, ovary, and breast
    b) Head and neck cancer
    c) Lymphomas
    d) Previous colorectal cancers
- *Streptococcus bovis* on blood culture (reason unknown)

These patients should be considered at very high risk for the development of carcinoma at an early age. Intense surveillance should be initiated, and referral may be required (see Referral section).

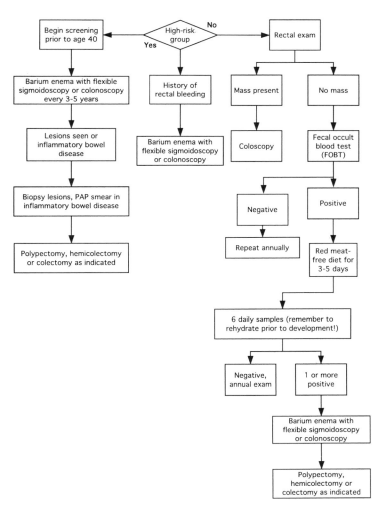

FIGURE 11-1. Algorithm for the management of colorectal screening.

Screening

Initial screening is done in two steps (see Figure 11-1): (1) rectal examination or rectovaginal exam for masses, and (2) fecal occult blood testing (FOBT). The rectovaginal exam is a fundamental component of the pelvic examination. Fecal occult blood testing, while inexpensive to perform, is controversial and its role in screening has recently been reviewed.[4] In a normal population the rate of false-positive results ranges from 1% to 4%.[5] False-negative results (patients with disease) may be as high as 50% because of the intermittent nature of bleeding in some lesions. The dilemma posed by false-positive test results and the resultant uncertainty about whether a more extensive work-up is indicated has yet to be resolved.[6] The high rate of false-positive results in patients under age 50 makes routine FOBT difficult to justify. A recent large prospective study has proved FOBT will reduce the mortality rate of colorectal cancer, but issues relating to cost effectiveness remain.[7] Despite objections over the utility of FOBT, however, there is no better screening test available, and the rate of morbidity and mortality from colorectal cancer remains high.

At the time of pelvic examination, a stool sample should be obtained and developed. Many false-positive results could be caused by the trauma to the cervix during the performance of the Pap test. The examining glove should be changed if obvious bleeding is evident. Another option is to give the patient FOBT cards and have 3–6 samples obtained and returned to the office for development. The samples should be rehydrated prior to applying developer. Because ingestion of red meat may result in false-positive results, a diet that is free of red meat should be consumed 3–5 days before testing.

Any positive test result is an indication for invasive diagnostic testing.

Some gynecologists have advocated the routine performance of flexible sigmoidoscopy as a screening method in patients over the age of 50. The American Gastrointestinal Society and the American Cancer Society (ACS) recommend that all patients over the age of 50 undergo sigmoidoscopy at 3- to 5-year intervals. The United States Preventative Services Task Force makes no recommendation for sigmoidoscopy. The benefit of routine sigmoidoscopy in colorectal cancer has never been proved. Ongoing assessments of outcomes underway in managed care environments may provide answers to questions regarding the benefit and cost effectiveness of this technique.

Diagnosis

Blood in the stool is the primary sign of colorectal cancer. In addition to colorectal cancer, a positive FOBT result could be caused by hemorrhoidal bleeding, red meat in the diet, and inflammatory and infectious diseases of the colon.

Rectal bleeding may be the first sign of bowel cancer; however, bleeding is not always associated with early lesions. Classic symptoms of bowel cancer usually are mechanical and are the result of partial obstructions. Low rectal carcinomas are associated with hematochezia, tenesmus, and narrowing of stool. Suggestive symptoms are abdominal pain, bloating, constipation, and diarrhea. Classically, bright red bleeding is associated with left-sided colonic lesions, whereas occult bleeding from the mixing of blood with stool occurs with right-sided lesions. The characteristic of the blood, either dark or clotted, has no clinical significance to location or prognosis.

Anemia, new onset of angina, increasing frequency of angina, heart failure, or general malaise and fatigue are presenting symptoms. Any postmenopausal patient who has iron deficiency anemia and no recent history of menometrorrhagia should be considered at high risk for carcinoma of the gastrointestinal tract. Barium studies of the upper gastrointestinal system (to investigate possible esophageal and gastric lesions), in addition to an assessment of the lower gastrointestinal tract, should be performed.

After a barium enema has been administered, flexible sigmoidoscopy can be performed to examine the first 25 cm of the rectum and sigmoid colon (the placement of the rectal catheter precludes adequate examination of this region). Two radiographic techniques of barium enema are available: (1) a single stream of barium, which is the easiest to perform and most comfortable for the patient; and (2) the air contrast technique, which has greater sensitivity but is time-consuming and uncomfortable for the patient. If a lesion is discovered, colonoscopy is performed to inspect the entire colon and biopsy suspicious lesions. For cost-containment purposes, many clinicians recommend colonoscopy instead of performing both a barium enema and a flexible sigmoidoscopy examination.[8] Carcinoembryonic antigen (CEA) is neither a screening nor a diagnostic test but is useful only as a means of monitoring disease activity.

Treatment

The primary goal in cancer treatment is the early detection and removal of lesions. Prognosis of colorectal carcinoma is directly related to size and penetration of lesions into underlying mucosa and tissues. The Dukes' classification is the most commonly used system:

A   Cancer limited to mucosa and submucosa
B   Cancer extends into muscularis or serosa of bowel wall
C   Regional lymph node involvement
D   Distant metastases (commonly lung, brain, liver, and su-
    praclavicular lymph nodes)

Staging is performed during surgical resection, and lymph node findings can be taken into consideration in the Dukes' classification. Mortality is directly related to the stage of disease at presentation. With the exception of lower rectal lesions, the only effective therapy for colon cancer is surgery. Lower rectal lesions respond to some extent to radiation. Anal carcinomas respond to both chemotherapy and radiation. Unfortunately, individuals with either advanced or recurrent disease respond poorly to adjunctive and salvage chemotherapies.

Referral

Patients who are at high risk of colorectal cancer because of associated diseases such as ulcerative colitis should be evaluated by a gastroenterologist. Patients with ulcerative colitis usually undergo yearly colonoscopy examination with Pap tests of lesions. When significant dysplasia arises in colonic lesions, total colectomy is recommended. Patients who have ulcerative colitis have a high incidence of malignant transformation after 15 years, especially if they are afflicted with pancolitis at a young age.

Individuals who are in high-risk groups require continuity of care and routine follow-up with endoscopy and are best cared for by a gastroenterologist. The basic evaluation should consist of either colonoscopy or barium enema with flexible sigmoidoscopy beginning at age 35 and continued at 3- to 5-year intervals.

► REFERENCES

1. Vogelstein B, Fearon ER, Hamilton SR, et al. Genetic alterations during colo-rectal-tumor development. *N Engl J Med* 1988;319:525–32.
2. Waillett WC, Stampfer MJ, Colditz GA, Rosner BA, Speizer FE. Relation of meat, fat, and fiber intake to the risk of colon cancer in a prospective study among women. *N Engl J Med* 1990;323:1664–72.
3. Burt RW, Bishop DT, Cannon LA, et al. Dominant inheritance of adenomatosis colonic polyps and colorectal cancer. *N Engl J Med* 1985;312:1540–4.
4. Toribara NW, Sleisenger MH. Current concepts: screening for colorectal can-cer. *N Engl J Med* 1995;332:861–7.
5. Lieberman DA. Colon cancer screening: the dilemma of positive screening tests. *Arch Intern Med* 1990;150:740–4.
6. Simon JB. Occult blood screening for colorectal carcinoma: a clinical review. *Gastroenterology* 1985;88:820–37.
7. Mandel JS, Bond JH, Church TR, et al. Reducing mortality from colorectal cancer by screening for occult blood. *N Engl J Med* 1993;328:1365–71.
8. Dasmahapatra KS, Lopyan K. Rationale for aggressive colonoscopy in patients with colorectal neoplasia. *Arch Surg* 1989;124:63–6.

GASTROINTESTINAL DISEASE

Diseases of the alimentary canal are common and, fortunately, usually not fatal. Chapter 12 focuses on the problems of acute diarrhea and all-too-common chronic constipation. Diarrhea is usually a self-limited disease and in many cases occurs secondary to food poisoning. Occasionally, diarrhea is secondary to malabsorption and systemic diseases such a Crohn's disease and ulcerative colitis. Irritable bowel syndrome may be confused with chronic pelvic pain and is a common problem in younger patients. Chapter 13 will deal with gallbladder disease, a frequent disease in women that may become more prevalent as more of the population becomes obese and hormonal replacement therapy more widespread. Gallbladder disease may be misdiagnosed because of vague symptoms and may present purely as frequent indigestion. The introduction of the use of ultrasound has eliminated low-yielding diagnostic tests such as oral cholecystography but has led to confusion concerning the management of asymptomatic women with gallstones.

Laparoscopic cholecystectomy has reduced postoperative morbidity but, as with other forms of laparoscopic surgery, has introduced a new set of complications.

Chapter 14 addresses the spectrum of peptic ulcer disease (PUD) and issues related to its management. Reflux esophagitis is a common malady that is easily treated but may be confused with cardiac chest pain and vice versa. The introduction of effective therapy with H_2 blockers and the release of these medications for over-the-counter use may lead to problems of self-diagnosis. Resistant cases of PUD may actually represent a missed diagnosis of gallbladder disease or erosive and potentially perforated ulcers. The role of the primary care physician as a diagnostician of upper abdominal complaints will be expanded in the managed care environment.

CHAPTER 12

Irritable Bowel Syndrome, Diarrhea, and Constipation

Disorders of the lower gastrointestinal tract can be chronic or acute. Certain disorders can be a cause of chronic pelvic pain and are often overlooked in a gynecologic assessment. The profile of patients affected by irritable bowel syndrome (IBS) and chronic pelvic pain is similar, and both conditions are linked to specific types of behavior. In the evaluation of chronic pelvic pain, a history directed toward irritable bowel syndrome should be obtained and, if present, treatment considered. Diarrhea can be chronic or acute and should be explored to detect underlying factors and related pathology. Constipation is often underdiagnosed in younger patients and may be a significant cause of chronic pelvic pain. Certain disorders of the gastrointestinal system are more prevalent in women and thus may first be evaluated by a gynecologist.

► IRRITABLE BOWEL SYNDROME

Irritable bowel syndrome is the most common gastrointestinal disorder encountered in a general medical practice. It is often overlooked as a cause of chronic pelvic pain in young patients.[1] Irritable bowel syndrome occurs twice as often in women as it does in men, and most patients are young to middle aged. The pathophysiology of IBS is unclear, but patients have altered motor reactivity to various stimuli, such as psychological stress and meals, which is related to bowel wall neural control mechanisms. Transit time in the gut is modified, resulting in pain, constipation, and diarrhea.

Screening

Functional gastrointestinal symptoms are common and affect up to 30% of patients. Three common clinical variants of IBS have been described:

1. "Spastic colitis," characterized by chronic abdominal pain and predominantly manifested by constipation.
2. Intermittent diarrhea (or, more accurately, multiple small stools), which is usually painless.
3. The classically described combination of alternating diarrhea and constipation.

Patients with IBS often exhibit behavioral patterns similar to those linked with chronic pelvic pain—hysteria, depression, and bipolar personality disorders. Because IBS has a large emotional overlay, the history is more important than physical examination. The patient should be asked about bowel function so symptoms can be related to certain stimuli. Irritable bowel syndrome is a diagnosis of exclusion that can be determined only after other disease states are eliminated based on the history.

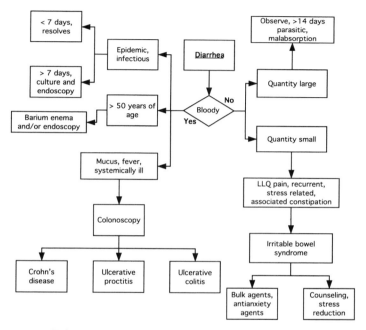

FIGURE 12-1. Algorithm for the assessment of diarrhea.

Diagnosis

Selected aspects of either the diarrhea or constipation algorithm (Figures 12-1 and 12-2) outline the diagnosis of IBS. A rectal examination should be performed. In the presence of a history of bloody stools, barium enema with sigmoidoscopy or colonoscopy should be performed to rule out pathologic changes. In younger patients, ulcerative colitis and Crohn's disease should be considered based on the presence of symp-

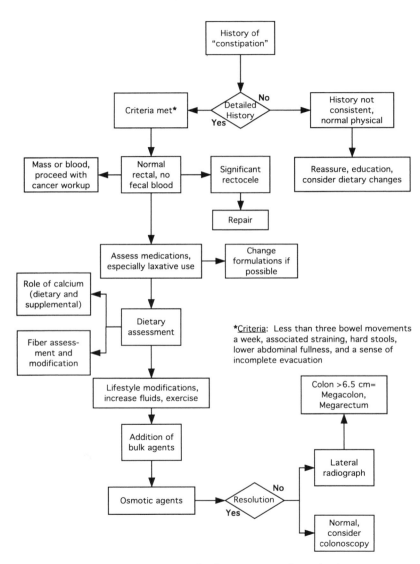

FIGURE 12-2. Algorithm for the assessment of constipation.

toms such as weight loss and bloody stools. In the rare older patient with symptoms of IBS, colorectal carcinoma should be considered. Most of these patients have no anatomic pathology, and diagnostic studies are usually of little value.

Treatment

Treatment of IBS is complicated by the underlying psychological problems that accompany many cases and the chronicity of the disorder.[2] After organic pathology has been excluded, psychological support, with emphasis on the chronic nature of the disorder, is important for long-term success.[3] Only if the patient's symptom complex significantly changes should further diagnostic studies be pursued. Most therapy is aimed at regulation of bowel function using bulk agents and increased dietary fiber. Patient education in many cases may be helpful for avoiding situations that induce stress and trigger symptoms. Mild sedation with phenobarbital and tranquilizers may afford some relief.

Referral

Many of these patients respond poorly to treatment and tend to seek care from numerous sources (sometimes in search of anti-anxiety medications). Many patients with IBS have poor outcomes, regardless of what is done, unless they acquire insight into the disease process and coping skills. Resistant cases should be referred to a gastroenterologist; in many cases the patient will self-refer to another physician.

▶ DIARRHEA

In The United States, diarrhea is the second most common illness after respiratory diseases. Diarrhea is most common in developing parts of the world because of poor food processing facilities and water sanitation. Internationally, acute diarrhea causes approximately 12,600 deaths per day, with the highest mortality in infants under the age of 5.[4]

Diarrhea is classified as acute or chronic. Acute diarrhea lasts less than 7–14 days, is usually self-limited, and commonly results from an infectious process. Chronic diarrhea lasts beyond 2–3 weeks and the cause may be either psychological or pathological. Acute diarrhea can be subdivided into different classes based on the presence or absence of blood in the stool and systemic illness. Chronic diarrhea syndromes are more commonly related to systemic diseases (Crohn's disease, ulcerative colitis, and celiac disease [nontropical sprue]), which are outside the scope of gynecologic practice.

Screening

In the developed world, diarrhea is defined as an increase in daily stool weight above 200 grams. Strict adherence to this criterion is necessary because individuals with IBS may have up to 10–12 bowel movements daily, but there is a small quantity of stool with each movement. Studies reported from the United Kingdom have shown that the average stool weight is approximately 55 g/day for females, which is one-third that of males.[5] Stool consistency has been difficult to quantitate because of a lack of standardization in liquid measurement; however, normal stool should not contain blood, white blood cells, parasites, fat, or muscle fibers.

History is the most important tool in evaluating diarrhea. Most patients with acute diarrhea seek care within 24–48 hours of the onset of symptoms. Abdominal pain with diarrhea should always be investigated for appendicitis, pelvic inflammatory disease, and adnexal torsion. Certain infectious agents may cause right lower-quadrant pain and can mimic appendicitis. Diagnostic laparoscopy should be used in questionable cases to evaluate peritoneal signs.

The complaint of "diarrhea" should be confirmed and not accepted as evidence that diarrhea is present. The number of normal bowel movements and the consistency should be determined. If a long history of IBS or "colitis" is suggested, a complete history of the size of stools and frequency of bowel movements should be obtained. Occasionally, fecal incontinence or incomplete evacuation is mistaken for diarrhea. The initial evaluation should focus on the following areas:

- *The acuteness or chronicity of the diarrhea.* If the patient has had diarrhea for more than 14 days and does not have obvious IBS, consultation is reasonable. Referral is indicated if there is a history of weight loss and chronicity.

- *The presence or absence of blood.* In younger patients with bloody diarrhea, the cause is usually an infectious agent, especially if there is a history of recent travel. In older patients ($>$50–55 years old), diarrhea may be the first (and only early) sign of colorectal cancer. A history of anorectal disorders (i.e., internal and external hemorrhoids, rectal fissures) can disclose important diagnostic possibilities. In the elderly, however, diarrhea should be assumed to be cancer until proved otherwise. Quantitating the amount of blood in the stool is difficult.

- *The presence or absence of systemic disease.* Symptoms such as anorexia, weight loss, fevers, fatigue, and chills may be indicative of inflammatory or neoplastic diseases. A long history of chronic diarrhea may be the result of lactose intolerance or celiac (nontropical sprue) disease. Referral to a gastroenterologist is probably prudent.

Nonbloody diarrhea in the absence of systemic symptoms is usually secondary to food poisoning, irritable bowel syndrome, lactose intolerance, or the use of various drugs. Diarrhea from contaminated food is rarely isolated to one individual but reported in clusters. Certain foods are commonly implicated: eggs, chicken products, and shellfish. Various organisms have been associated with particular time sequences after exposure (Table 12-1). In most outbreaks, affected groups become ill within 24–36 hours of exposure. Other causes of acute nonbloody diarrhea are the use of antibiotics or magnesium-containing antacids (surreptitious cathartic use is common in chronic laxative abusers with self-treated "constipation"). Sorbitol, which is found in sugarless chewing gum, and fructose in diet drinks may be responsible. Lactose intolerance can be familial and is common in African–Americans and Asians. Diarrhea follows the consumption of diary products, especially milk and ice cream.

Drinking of contaminated water sources, especially from fresh streams in western mountain areas, should raise suspicion for giardiasis. Contact with children, especially if they are in a child care environment, may cause diarrhea in adults.

Acute onset of bloody diarrhea in the absence of systemic illness should raise suspicion of colorectal carcinoma, even in the young. Rectal bleeding may be the first sign of diverticulosis, ulcerative colitis, or proctitis. Ulcerative colitis is

▶ **TABLE 12-1   Sources of Food Contamination and Onset of Symptoms**

Less than 6 Hours

Staphylococcus aureus: Commonly found in mayonnaise, especially in potato and egg salad, ham, and poultry

Bacillus cereus: Common in fried rice (when symptom onset is of this short a duration)

8–16 Hours

Bacillus cereus: Found in meats, vegetables, and cereals (with this longer duration of symptom onset)

Clostridium perfringens: Common in gravies, poultry, and beef

Greater than 16 Hours

Enterotoxigenic *E. coli*: A variety of sources including water, meats, cheese, and salads

Vibrio cholerae: Shellfish, usually from contaminated beds

Vibrio parahaemolyticus: Found in crustaceans and shellfish

Salmonella: Common in eggs and dairy products; less common in beef and poultry

Shigella: Found in raw vegetable, potato, and egg salads

associated with systemic illness, fatigue, and weight loss. If the blood appears on toilet paper and is of scant quantity, hemorrhoids may be the cause. Recurrent blood in the stool or on toilet tissue warrants more extensive evaluation. Bloody diarrhea in a systemically ill patient is usually caused by secondary inflammatory bowel disease (Crohn's disease, ulcerative colitis) and infectious agents (most commonly bacterial and parasitic).

Bacterial diseases commonly associated with bloody diarrhea include *Shigella, Salmonella, Campylobacter,* and *Yersinia* species. Additionally, pathologic forms of *Escherichia coli* may be responsible. Pseudomembranous colitis may be associated with recent antibiotic use but is rare in individuals taking long-term antibiotic therapy, such as tetracycline use for acne. Recent travel or epidemics among family members or social groups suggest a bacterial pathogen.

Diagnosis

For acute outbreaks, the history usually confirms the diagnosis. The routine use of cultures in the diagnosis of bacterial agents is rarely helpful and thus discouraged. Cultures may be required, however, to diagnose cases of bloody diarrhea that persist more than a few days. If systemic illness is present or colorectal carcinoma suspected, a diagnostic work-up (including barium enema with flexible sigmoidoscopy or colonoscopy) is indicated.

Treatment

Most cases of diarrhea are self-limited and should be treated with adequate hydration and observation. "Traveler's diarrhea" has become more common in the United States with the advent of cheaper airfares to Mexico and Latin America. The frequent use of broad spectrum antibiotics in these regions is discouraged because of evolving resistant bacterial species. A nonantibiotic regimen should be considered first and should be prescribed prior to travel. If giardiasis is suspected (on the basis of mobile trophozoites identified in a stool sample by wet preparation), a 1-week course of metronidazole (250 mg three times daily) is indicated. Diverticulitis should be treated with intravenous broad spectrum antibiotics.

Referral

The history determines whether the patient should be treated by a gynecologist or referred to a gastroenterologist. Patients with chronic diarrhea and malabsorption problems require extensive evaluation. If polyps are identified during routine sigmoidoscopy, removal may require an experienced practitioner. Any suspicious lesions identified by barium enema usually should be evaluated with colonoscopy. Systemically ill individuals with bloody diarrhea may require evaluation by a gastroenterologist to rule out inflammatory bowel disease. If inflammatory bowel disease is diagnosed, the patient should be referred to a gastroenterologist for long-term management.

▶ CONSTIPATION

Complaints of "constipation" may be secondary to infrequent stools, difficult bowel movements, bloating, or incomplete evacuation.[6] Constipation is more common in individuals over the age of 65. It is not limited to the elderly, however, and is often underdiagnosed in young women. Few studies have addressed "normal" intervals of bowel movements based on age. Laxative use increases in elderly individuals and may contribute to "normal" stool frequency.

Constipation, by strict definition, is described as having fewer than three bowel movements weekly, but individual variation should be taken into consideration. The most important aspect of evaluating constipation is not the frequency of stooling but rather the associated symptoms of painful defecation or bloating. Decrease in bowel frequency, especially in the elderly, may be related to decreased motility in the anorectal region.

This condition, termed dyschezia, is failure of the puborectalis of the pelvic diaphragm to relax during defecation attempts.

Screening

Multiple drugs are associated with altered bowel function, and an extended history of related causes (e.g., use of over-the-counter medications) should be obtained. Antacids containing aluminum hydrazide and calcium carbonate are commonly ingested drugs that induce constipation. Anticholinergic medications and antidepressants (especially tricyclics) are frequently implicated. Calcium channel-blocking agents, especially verapamil, are well known to cause severe constipation. Iron, in therapeutic doses, contributes to hard stools. Narcotic agents, nonsteroidal anti-inflammatory drugs, and sympathomimetics (pseudoephedrine commonly added to combat sedation in cold preparations) also may result in difficult bowel movements. A detailed medication profile, with special emphasis on over-the-counter drugs, including calcium chloride tablets for heartburn and cold preparations, should be sought.

Hypothyroidism is a common cause of altered bowel function, especially in the presence of a family history of thyroid disorders. Thyroid replacement therapy should reverse this process. Other causes of constipation include long-standing insulin-dependent diabetes (especially with gastroparesis), neuropathy of any etiology, scleroderma, Parkinson's disease, and hypercalcemia from malignancy.

Patient age and the rapidity of onset of symptoms are important factors in determining the etiology. Sudden changes in stooling such as change in caliber of stool, intermittent diarrhea, or bloody stool should be evaluated for carcinoma of the colon. Colorectal cancer usually is detected in patients over the age of 50, but a certain subset of patients may develop symptoms in their teens.[7] Colorectal cancer occurs equally among men and women. Certain families are at higher risk, and certain medical conditions (i.e., ulcerative colitis, familial polyposis) contribute to increased risk.[8]

Hirschsprung's disease, a condition limited to the colon that can cause constipation, often is first diagnosed in children but may occur at any age. Other conditions that may result in severe constipation include idiopathic megarectum and megacolon. These diseases of undetermined etiology are associated with a dilated rectum without distal-narrowed colonic segments. Severe constipation often occurs accompanied by intermittent abdominal pain associated with distention. Interestingly, many of these patients have normal anorectal reflexes.[9]

Diagnosis

Physical examination yields little information in most cases. An exception is patients with tympanitic bowel sounds or with large masses secondary to retained stool or tumor mass. Digital examination of the rectum may differentiate between rectal diseases (masses, large quantities of hard stool) and colonic diseases (minimal stool in the vault). If it is necessary to document abnormal gut motility, stool transit time should be assessed. Twenty radiopaque markers (these may be made by cutting up a nasogastric tube) are ingested daily for 3 days. On days 4 and 7 plain abdominal films are obtained. The number of markers in the right and left colon and rectosigmoid are counted and multiplied times 1.2 to determine the transit time in hours for each colonic segment. Normal range is from 35 to 72 hours.[10]

A lateral radiograph revealing a rectal diameter of more than 6.5 cm at the pelvic brim can establish the diagnosis of megacolon and megarectum. If the suspected cause of megarectum or megacolon is cancer, water-soluble rather than lipid-soluble dyes should be used to prevent barium impactions. Anorectal physiology studies to measure muscle contractions are available and should be considered only if the individual does not respond to dietary changes and other simple maneuvers. If laxative abuse is suspected, flexible sigmoidoscopy may reveal pigment changes in colonic mucosa referred to as *melanosis coli*. This unique discoloration is confirmatory of laxative abuse of the anthraquinone class (cascara and senna).

Treatment

Accurate diagnosis is important in treating constipation. Treatment of an underlying medical disease, such as hypothyroidism, usually will relieve related constipation. Likewise, if constipation is induced by medication, changing the medication or discontinuing its use is effective.

Bowel training is important in patients of all ages. Patients should be instructed to attempt a bowel movement daily, either in the morning or in the evening. Mornings and evenings are chosen because it is the most effective time for augmentation of the gastrocolic reflex. In elderly patients, the gastrocolic reflex is critical because of a decrease in the defecation reflex. Attempts should be made for a minimum of 10 undistracted minutes, usually in the morning.

Regular exercise, especially in the elderly, may help relieve constipation.[11] Physical exercise stimulates the gastrointestinal tract and may increase fluid intake. An exercise program, tailored to limitations such as visual problems to prevent falls and fractures, should be recommended. In many patients fast walking is all that is necessary to stimulate normal bowel function.

Increased consumption of fiber is advocated for good health and may reverse constipation. Dietary fiber may be purchased as a pill supplement in health food stores. Fiber may worsen some problems, primarily bloating and gas. Fluid intake should be increased in general and, if taken with fiber medication, by at least 1 glass of water for each dose.

If life-style changes do not alter the frequency of bowel movements, laxatives may be necessary. Laxative use may have been initiated by the patient. All medications should be reviewed and, if possible, substituted or eliminated. The type of laxative used and its effectiveness should be documented prior to initiating therapy. Laxatives are divided into five major categories based on either their mechanism of action or chemical grouping: bulk agents, saline, hyperosmotics, stimulants, and emollients.

Bulk agents include bran, methyl cellulose, wheat husk, and psyllium derivatives. The ease of administration and the over-the-counter availability of these agents contribute to their popularity. Most agents are hydrophilic and increase stool mass while softening the stool. Flatulence and abdominal distention are distressing side effects, but these effects eventually resolve.

Commonly used hyperosmolar agents include saline laxatives, milk of magnesia, magnesium citrate, and sodium phosphate enemas. Use of these compounds results in active fluid secretion from the wall of the colon into the gut lumen. Saline laxatives are often used as preprocedural bowel preparations.

These agents are not suitable for long-term use but rather should be reserved for episodic use when bulk and other agents are unsuccessful. Lactulose is a semisynthetic disaccharide laxative that has been actively promoted for patients with constipation. The product never became popular in the United States because it required frequent dosage intervals (three or four times daily) and quantities (30 mL/dose).

Emollients or stool softeners such as dioctyl sodium sulfosuccinate (Colace) and mineral oil are bulk agents that are useful in the elderly. The mode of action is to incorporate water into the stool mass, which also softens fecal material. Additionally, after metabolism by the enterohepatic circulation, bulk agents stimulate the colon. Glycerin suppositories lubricate the anorectal area and stimulate the defecation reflex when inserted.

Stimulant laxatives directly stimulate the myenteric plexus of the colon. There are two representative classes of these commonly used preparations: the anthraquinone derivatives (aloe, senna, and cascara) and polyphenolic derivatives. These agents should only be used episodically because of their ability to cause permanent damage to the myenteric plexuses, resulting in refractory constipation. Unfortunately, this class of medications is abused regularly, resulting in a vicious cycle of increasing doses, which may finally result in permanent damage. Castor oil inhibits glucose and sodium absorption while stimulating water and electrolyte secretion. When used in large quantities, it may lead to serious fluid and electrolyte disturbances. Bisacodyl (Ducolax) remains with the lumen of the gut and has a direct stimulatory effect on the myenteric plexus. With large doses, diarrhea with hypokalemia and salt overload may result. Stimulative laxatives should only be used as a last resort rather than as a primary mode of therapy.

Referral

The presence of recurrent obstipation, especially in the elderly, requires a work-up of colorectal carcinoma. Megacolon or megarectum are difficult problems to manage and should be referred to a gastroenterologist. If simple maneuvers such as diet or the addition of bulk agents and emollients are unresponsive, long-term management by a gastroenterologist is warrented.

▶ REFERENCES

1. Longstreth GF. Irritable bowel syndrome and chronic pelvic pain. *Obstet Gynecol Surv* 1994;49:505–7.

2. Mitchell CM, Drossman DA. The irritable bowel syndrome: understanding and treating a biopsychosocial illness disorder. *Ann Behav Med* 1987;9:13–8.

3. Drossman DA, Thompson WG. The irritable bowel syndrome: review and a graduated multicomponent treatment approach. *Ann Intern Med* 1992;116: 1009–16.

4. Guerrant RL, Hughes JM, Lima NL, Crane J. Diarrhea in developed and developing countries: magnitude, special settings, and etiologies. *Rev Infect Dis* 1990;12:S41–50.

5. Schiller LR, Hogan RB, Morawski SG, et al. Studies of the prevalence and significance of radiolabelled bile acid malabsorption in a group of patients with idiopathic chronic diarrhea. *Gastroenterology* 1987;92:151–60.

6. Hinton JM, Lennard-Jones JE. Constipations: definition and classification. *Postgrad Med J* 1968;44:720–3.

7. Steinberg JB, Tuggle DW, Postier RG. Adenocarcinoma of the colon in adolescents. *Am J Surg* 1988;156:460–2.

8. Nolan TE. Colorectal cancer: the gynecologist's role. *Female Patient* 1991;16:18A–H.

9. Gattuso JM, Kamm MA. Review article: the management of constipation in adults. *Aliment Pharmacol Ther* 1993;7:487–500.

10. Hinton JM, Lennard-Jones JE, Young AC. A new method of studying gut transit times using radio-opaque markers. *Gut* 1969;8:42–7.

11. Holdstock DJ, Misiewicz JJ, Smith T, et al. Propulsion (mass movements) in the human colon: its relationship to meals and somatic activity. *Gut* 1970;11:91–9.

CHAPTER 13

Gallbladder Disease

Gallbladder disease affects 2 million people—approximately 10% of the population—annually in the United States, resulting in an estimated one-half million surgical procedures. The incidence of gallbladder disease is three times greater in women than in men, so an awareness of its presentations and treatment modalities is essential.

History

Although gallbladder disease can occur at any age, 70% of patients are over the age of 40, and age along represents one of the major risk factors. Estrogen (both natural and pharmacologic) affects solubility factors that contribute to the formation of gallstones.[1] Obesity is also a recognized risk factor. As weight increases, so does the incidence of cholelithiasis: individuals 15–20 lb overweight have a twofold increase in risk, and an excess of 50–75 lb increases the risk sixfold.[2] Interestingly, rapid weight loss also increases the risk of cholelithiasis. Other conditions that increase risk include cirrhosis, diabetes, and Crohn's disease. A family history of cholelithiasis in siblings or children increases risk twofold. Finally, American Indians and Mexican–Americans are at greater risk of developing disease.

An altered cholesterol/bile acid ratio increases the risk of precipitation and is the most common cause of cholelithiasis. Cholesterol stone formation may also occur when bilirubin concentrations are increased, such as in hemolysis anemia. Biliary stasis further increases the risk of cholesterol precipitation, causing stone formation. Biliary stasis occurs for many reasons such as mechanical changes in the biliary tree or dietary or hormonal factors. Once a small stone is formed, it may acquire further layers of cholesterol, mucin, and bilirubin salts, growing until it is detectable and causes symptoms. Once this occurs, cholelithiasis enters the clinical stages. The following high-risk factors should be considered in the evaluation of gallbladder disease:

- Age > 40
- Sex (female/male = 3:1)
- Pregnancy
- Oral contraceptive use
- Oral estrogen replacement
- Obesity
- Diet and medications
- Cirrhosis
- Diabetes
- Crohn's disease
- Family history

Diagnosis

The clinical progression of cholelithiasis is variable. Although 4% of patients with gallstones remain asymptomatic, 50% of asymptomatic patients will eventually develop symptoms and 20% will experience severe complications. Common symptoms include dyspepsia, fatty food intolerance, biliary colic, and, rarely, jaundice. Biliary colic results from intermittent obstruction of the biliary tree and presents as right upper-quadrant, midepigastric, or subscapular pain; nausea; or vomiting. Fever may be a sign of ascending cholangitis, a medical–surgical emergency. Jaundice, which may be confused with hepatitis, is rare and occurs when the common duct is obstructed. Additionally, the jaundice may be elusive if a stone is passed. The most common complication of gallbladder disease is acute cholecystitis. Anatomically, obstructions usually occur in the neck of the gallbladder or the cystic bile duct. Untreated, obstructions may result in ischemia and gangrene of the gallbladder. Vomiting is present in 75% of patients and may resolve in 12–18 hours if the obstruction is transient. Symptoms are often mistaken for indigestion. Acute cholecystitis may lead to chronic cholecystitis, with repeated attacks of varying degrees. Cholangitis, or inflammation in the bile-collecting system by an enteric organism, is associated with colicky pain, fever, and jaundice. Untreated, the infected gallbladder can cause significant morbidity and mortality.

Pregnancy increases the risk of cholelithiasis, especially in association with multiple pregnancies and rising parity. After appendectomy, cholecystectomy represents the second most common surgery performed during pregnancy. Symptoms of cholelithiasis develop in 4% of pregnant women. Cholestasis occurring during pregnancy produces variable symptoms, ranging from mild pruritus to jaundice. Stones are the cause of 5–9% of cases of jaundice in pregnancy. Cholestasis usually occurs in the last one-half of pregnancy and progresses until after delivery, when it resolves. Of those women who enter pregnancy with known gallstones, 40% become symptomatic and 31% develop symptoms postpartum. Fewer than 3% of patients with cholelithiasis during pregnancy undergo surgery. Fetal mortality approaches 5% with surgery and increases to 60% with coexisting pancreatitis.

Pancreatitis is a serious complication of gallstone disease, and cholelithiasis should be considered in cases of acute illness. Approximately 50% of cases of pancreatitis are secondary to biliary tract disease. Cancer of the gallbladder is a rare complication of cholelithiasis, occurring in 0.2–5% of patients. Unfortunately, it is insidious in onset and usually presents as painless jaundice.

Laboratory evaluation is supportive and may suggest but not confirm the diagnosis. Liver function tests should be performed, especially when jaundice is present. An elevated serum bilirubin level may be useful in diagnosing obstruction, and an elevated serum amylase value may indicate, but is not diagnostic of, pancreatitis. A high serum alkaline phosphatase level may indicate obstruction, but levels also may be elevated because of pregnancy. Elevated serum transaminase values (SGOT or SGPT) can indicate altered metabolic function related to damage from obstruction.

The standard tool used to diagnose cholelithiasis is abdominal ultrasonography, which is 96% accurate in diagnosing sludge or a stone. Ultrasonography has essentially replaced oral cholecystography as the diagnostic test of choice. The rate of false-negative results with oral cholecystography is high, and 20% of patients experience nausea, vomiting, or diarrhea from the contrast agent. Only 20% of stones have sufficient calcium for accurate imaging with abdominal flat-plate roentgenography. Nucleotide imaging (HIDA scans) may be useful for the diagnosis of acute cholelithiasis but cannot detect stones in asymptomatic patients. Endoscopic retrograde cholangiopancreatography (ERCP) (i.e., the cannulation of the ampulla of Vater through endoscopy with dye injection), intravenous cholangiography, and transhepatic cholangiography are useful only for selected acute cases and are not suitable for routine screening or testing.

Treatment

Controversy exists over the need for surgical treatment of asymptomatic or rarely symptomatic gallstones. However, complications of cholelithiasis markedly increase the risk of emergency surgery, resulting in a dramatic increase in the risk of morbidity and mortality.

Management of cholelithiasis depends on a number of factors, including patient and physician preference. Variables to be considered in selecting therapy include the severity and character of symptoms, stone composition and size, and availability of various treatment modalities. In some patients, dietary modification aimed at reducing cholesterol and fatty food intake may decrease the frequency and severity of recurrences. This expectant management probably will not alter the progression of symptoms over time, however, because spontaneous reabsorption of existing gallstones is rare.

Depending on the size and character of the stones, oral therapy may be an option. Chenodeoxycholic acid has been used to shrink cholesterol stones; however, even high doses may produce limited results. Another new oral agent is ursodeoxycholic acid, which increases the solubility of cholesterol in bile by promoting the formation of a lecithin–cholesterol liquid layer on the stone surface. This agent has been very effective in decreasing the size of cholesterol gallstones over time without an adverse impact on serum lipid or cholesterol levels. The rate of a stone's dissolution (approximately 1 mm per month) limits the applicability of this therapy to stones less than 1.5–2 cm in size. Fortunately, most gallstones are smaller than this. Oral therapy has had a favorable effect on resorption of cholesterol stones, with resolution of symptoms in 2–3 months. Unfortunately, 50% of patients experience a recurrence of stones after cessation of therapy.[3]

Surgery remains the definitive therapy for gallstones. Cholecystectomy ranks second only to endoscopy in the frequency of digestive system surgery. Surgical complications are common, with 0.7–1.2% mortality in asymptomatic patients, rising to almost 5% in the presence of acute cholangitis or pancreatitis. When surgery involves common duct exploration, the risk of complications triples. The risk of surgery also increases with age. Interestingly, complications are less common in women than in men.

Endoscopic sphincterotomy has been employed in the past to remove stones up to 1–1.5 cm. Its use is restricted to stones in the common duct. Although this procedure has a 90% success rate, it also has a 10% rate of major complications and a 1–1.5% mortality rate. Similarly, percutaneous extraction of gallstones via a tube tract has not been successful in replacing standard cholecystectomy.

Laparoscopy has become the primary approach to cholecystectomy, and the performance of "open" surgery has decreased. Two large trocars are positioned (one umbilical and one midline midway between the umbilicus and subxiphoid), followed by two or three abdominal punctures in the right subcostal area to allow dissection with laser, cautery, and clips. Variability of anatomy poses some operative problems. Cholangiography is technically formidable and common duct stones or common duct disease may be overlooked with laparoscopy. Complications occur in about 5% of cases and include bleeding from the cystic artery or liver bed, bile leakage, or damage to the common duct. Recent studies report a 5% conversion from laparoscopy to conventional surgery because of unexpected findings or problems. Reductions in cost, operating time, hospital stay, and postoperative morbidity are the main advantages of laparoscopy.[4]

Lithotripsy, first popularized in the treatment of ureteral lithiasis, can be applied to gallstone dissolution. Lithotripsy mechanically disrupts the stone but has no effect on resorption. Many physicians combine lithotripsy with oral therapy to hasten absorption and decrease the possibility of small fragments becoming a nidus for further stone growth. Success with this combined approach has been good. Overall efficacy of this technique is less dependent on stone composition than other techniques, but it is best suited to patients with no more than three large stones. Additionally, candidates for lithotripsy must also have normal liver and gallbladder function and not have acute disease.

Contraindications to lithotripsy are age less than 18 years, more than three stones, or stones greater than 3 cm. Obesity is a relative contraindication. Side effects are petechiae in 14% of patients and hematuria in 3% of patients. The most common complication of lithotripsy is biliary colic, which occurs in 35% of patients. Overall, lithotripsy has not been as popular for cholelithiasis as it is for ureterolithiasis, especially with the advent of laparoscopic surgery.[4]

Referral

The role of the obstetrician–gynecologist in the management of gallbladder disease is usually diagnostic and not therapeutic. Medical therapy in most cases is usually limited to patients with severe and multiple medical complications. Because of recurrence rates, surgical approaches are usually recommended, and laparoscopy has become more available and commonly used for this procedure.

▶ REFERENCES

1. Boston Collaborative Drug Surveillance Program: surgically confirmed gallbladder disease, venous thromboembolism, and breast tumors in relation to postmenopausal estrogen therapy. *N Engl J Med* 1974;290:15–9.
2. Everson GT, McKinley C, Kern F Jr. Mechanisms of gallstone formation in women. *J Clin Invest* 1991;87:237–46.
3. Fromm H. Gallstone dissolution therapy. Current status and future prospects. *Gastroenterology* 1986;91:1560–7.
4. Southern Surgeons Club. A prospective analysis of 1518 laparoscopic cholecystectomies. *N Engl J Med* 1991;324;1073–8.

CHAPTER 14

Gastric Disorders

Gastric acid is essential to the breakdown and digestion of complex foodstuffs to smaller molecules that are then absorbed. Because acid is necessary in the process of absorption, the stomach possesses protective mechanisms against the erosive effects of acid. When acid is in contact with other organs or when defense barriers are compromised, damage may occur. Two such examples are gastroesophageal reflux disease (GERD), or "heartburn," in which esophageal tissues are irritated by stomach acids, and peptic ulcer disease (PUD), in which the mucosa of the stomach and duodenum are damaged by peptic acid.

► GASTROESOPHAGEAL REFLUX

Reflux of gastric acid on sensitive esophageal tissues may result in substernal chest pain. This chest pain may radiate to the neck and be confused with cardiac chest pain. Certain myocardial infarctions (inferior wall) may be associated with "severe heartburn" and be misdiagnosed, especially by the patient. Therefore, any chest pain syndrome that is atypical or consistent with the pattern and distribution of cardiac symptoms requires immediate evaluation and referral.[1]

179

History

Heartburn is the cardinal manifestation of GERD. The most common cause of heartburn is the retrograde movement of acid from the stomach to the columnar-lined, sensitive esophagus.[2] Usually this occurs as a result of decreased tone in lower esophageal sphincter (LES) pressure. The following factors are associated with GERD:

- Obesity and pregnancy
- Girdles, abdominal binders
- Foods: fatty foods, chocolate, high-acid content (citric juice)
- Carminative substances: onion, garlic, and peppermint
- Cigarette smoking
- Calcium channel blockers
- Nonsteroidal anti-inflammatory agents
- Progestins in high doses

Diagnosis

Symptoms usually occur after consuming large meals, eating certain foods, and lying down. In contrast to the burning pain characteristic of dyspepsia, motor disorders of the esophagus, such as achalasia or muscular spasm ("nutcracker" esophagus), usually have symptoms of regurgitation and severe chest pain syndromes. Prolonged esophageal exposure to acid may lead to stricture formation and, eventually, dysphagia. Fortunately, strictures are rare, but affected patients experience prolonged periods of chest pain. Nocturnal aspiration may be more common than thought because it is silent, resulting in laryngitis and, in extreme cases, wheezing that may be mistaken for asthma. Erosive esophagitis from chronic reflux may lead to subclinical bleeding and iron deficiency anemia.

After a careful history to confirm that the symptom complex is consistent with mild disease (absence of acute abdomen, longevity of symptoms), empiric therapy may be initiated in patients with uncomplicated GERD. Patients with anemia, excessive weight loss, symptoms consistent with pulmonary aspiration (sudden awakening with cough, choking, wheezing, or laryngospasm), and dysphagia should undergo further evaluation prior to starting medication.

Initial diagnostic studies include either air-contrast barium study or upper gastrointestinal endoscopy. The air-contrast barium study is less sensitive than endoscopy, whereas endoscopy is more sensitive but also more expensive. Determination of the best test should be guided by clinical presentation; for example, weight loss and anemia could indicate cancer and are best evaluated by endoscopy. These studies can be used to eliminate other potential causes of GERD, including esophageal motility disorders, erosive esophagitis, and peptic ulcer disease (gastric or duodenal) (Figure 14-1).

Treatment

Life-style adjustments are as important as medication in overall management. Cigarette smoking should be stopped because it lowers LES pressure and delays esophageal acid clearance, increasing acid exposure to the esophageal mucosa. Patients should not lie down for 2–3 hours after consuming a large meal because postural changes (recumbency, bending over) contribute to LES relaxation and reflux. Placing the head of the

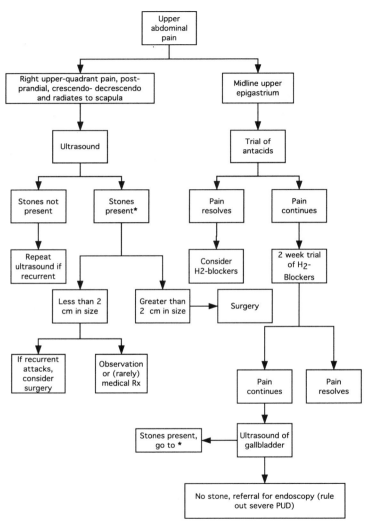

FIGURE 14-1. Algorithm for upper abdominal pain.

patient's bed on 6–8 inch blocks or using a bed wedge decreases acid exposure time and is as effective as medication in healing reflux esophagitis.[3] Foods with high acid content, such as orange juice, should be eliminated from the patient's diet. Fatty foods and chocolate have the dual effects of decreasing LES pressure and delaying gastric emptying. Carminatives are naturally occurring substances found in onions, garlic, peppermint, and certain after-dinner liquors. These foods increase gas, cause belching, and lower LES pressure.

Pharmacologic therapy should be initiated only after lifestyle adjustments are instituted. Prior to initiating therapy, the use of medications that reduce LES pressure (anticholinergics, diazepam, and calcium channel blockers) or those that contribute to direct damage to the esophageal mucosa (NSAIDs) should be discontinued if possible. Antacids were once the drug of choice in the treatment of GERD; however, frequent dosing intervals of 1 and 3 hours after meals and at bedtime result in poor compliance. Antacid preparations contain varying amounts of inorganic salts, which may cause diarrhea, bloating, or constipation and limit compliance. Antacids are cheap and readily available, however, and may be used in mild disease. They may be useful in the initial assessment of pain disorders, such as cardiac chest pain.

With the introduction in the mid-1970s of H_2-antagonists, which interfere with gastric acid production, treatment of GERD and peptic ulcer disease changed dramatically. Cimetidine, ranitidine, and famotidine are common medications in this class and may be prescribed in various doses and intervals, depending on disease symptoms and severity.

For GERD, cimetidine (200 mg), ranitidine (150 mg), and famotidine (20 mg) may be prescribed at bedtime. Currently, the U.S. Food & Drug Administration is evaluating these medications for over-the-counter use. Omeprazole is a new medication that inhibits the gastric hydrogen–potassium pump, neutralizing stomach acid. Because data on long-term use are not available, this medication should be used for only 8–12 weeks.

Referral

Patients who are resistant to H_2-antagonists should be referred for more aggressive therapy and work-up, which includes antireflux surgery. Other causes of abdominal pain should be considered such as pancreatitis and gallbladder disease. The primary care physician should consider an ultrasound if the pain is atypical. Most patients will require endoscopy prior to surgery to interrupt the vagus nerve.

▶ PEPTIC ULCER DISEASE

Peptic ulcer disease (PUD) is caused by acid and pepsin damage to the mucosa of the stomach and duodenum after disruption of normal host factors. Peptic ulcer disease may be the result of either an increase in acid and pepsin production or a breakdown of defenses. Control or alteration of peptic acid secretion is the cornerstone of therapy for PUD. Secretion of peptic acid is controlled by three endogenous chemicals: (1) acetylcholine, which is released when the vagus nerve is stimulated; (2) gastrin, which is released by protein in food; and (3) histamine, which is secreted by mastlike cells via a paracrine (local release of endocrine substances into adjacent cells) mechanisms.[4]

To counter the effect of these potentially destructive chemicals, three levels of defense are postulated to protect gastric and duodenal mucosa:

1. Surface epithelial cells secrete a mucus and bicarbonate substance, creating a protective barrier for the mucosa.
2. A neutral pH is present at the mucosal level, allowing an acid environment in the lumen of the stomach or intestine.
3. Blood flow to the mucosa in the gastrointestinal tract is extensive, quickly removing acid from the mucosal epithelium.

An additional protective factor is the rapid cell renewal process that constantly goes on in the entire gut, replacing damaged and sloughed cells. Endogenous prostaglandins (PGE_1, PGE_2) enhance cellular renewal and increase mucus production, bicarbonate production, and blood flow. Disruption of prostaglandin production may therefore be important in the genesis of peptic ulcer disease.

History

Despite an apparent link between gastrin secretion and gastric ulcers, most patients with gastric ulcers have low-to-normal levels of gastrin. A hereditary link has been described in patients with multiple endocrine neoplasm syndrome and other rare syndromes such as Zollinger–Ellison syndrome. Little evidence supports a genetic basis for PUD; however, a three times higher incidence is found among first-degree relatives with duodenal ulcer. Up to 40% of patients have an increased secretion rate of acid but most patients have normal rates of acid secretion.

Breakdown of the mucosal barrier is probably the single most important factor in peptic ulcer disease. Definite factors associated with the disruption of the mucosal barrier include (1) infection with *Helicobacter pylori,* (2) cigarette smoking, and (3) use of NSAIDs including aspirin. Etiologic agents such as alcohol use, stress, and adrenocorticosteroids are now considered less important. The association of *H. pylori* infection and PUD has been controversial. Arguments to support its role in PUD are compelling: *H. pylori* has been isolated in 95% of patients with duodenal ulcers and in 70% of patients with gastric ulcers. Individuals accidentally exposed to *H. pylori* have become ill with acute symptomatic gastritis. *Helicobacter pylori* is associated with inflammation and disruption of the mucosal barrier, which allows further disruption by acid and pepsin.[5]

Cigarette smoking is associated with increased acid formation, alteration in blood flow, and interference with prostaglandin production. NSAIDs have a direct effect on the disruption of the mucosal barrier, ranging from superficial lesions to deep ulceration.[6]

Diagnosis

Symptoms of PUD, such as dyspepsia, represent a broad constellation of complaints and disorders. In addition to pain in the upper abdomen, associated symptoms include nausea, vomiting, anorexia, fullness, and bloating. Pain may be described as cramping, gnawing, or burning anywhere in the upper abdomen. Pain may be elusive and of short duration. Response to meals is variable, and the correlation between symptoms and demonstrated ulcers is poor. Physical examination is rarely helpful, except when serious complications such as perforation or obstruction result in an acute abdomen.

Useful diagnostic tests are either radiographic studies or esophagogastroduodenoscopy. Radiographic studies may miss up to 20% of ulcers, which may account for the widespread popularity of endoscopy. Direct visualization of ulcers and erosions is possible and, if carcinoma is suspected, direct biopsies may be performed. In some cases, neither diagnostic test may identify an ulcer, despite the presence of classic symptoms (pain disappearing with food or antacids). This condition is referred to as nonulcer dyspepsia and the patient should be offered a trial of therapy.

Treatment

Several therapies are effective in treating ulcers. Ulcers usually require a minimum of 12 weeks of therapy to heal. Antacids, once a mainstay of therapy, are used less often because of the need for frequent dosing and common agent-dependent side effects of diarrhea (magnesium hydroxide) or constipation (aluminum hydroxide). If antacids are used, a low-sodium formulation should be considered. Anticholinergic drugs, another group of drugs commonly used in the past, are rarely used now because they are ineffective in accelerating healing and have troublesome side effects of blurred vision and dry mouth. Antisecretory agents, including H_2-receptor antagonists (cimetidine, ranitidine, and famotidine), are the most common medications used in the treatment of ulcer disease.[7] Currently, manufacturers are applying for over-the-counter status for these compounds. These agents have been successfully used for years with infrequent side effects and a high degree of patient compliance.

▶ **TABLE 14-1   Therapy for *H. pylori* Infections**

Double Therapy	Triple Therapy
Amoxicillin 1 gram bid with omeprazole 20 mg bid for 2 weeks	Two tablets of Pepto-Bismol with 500 mg tetracycline and 250 mg metronidazole qid with meals and at bedtime for 2 weeks
Cure rate 60–80%	Cure rate 85–95%
Costs ≥ $125	Costs $40–50
Compliance much better; however, if initiation of antibiotics is delayed, therapy is less effective	Compliance an issue; diarrhea noted in up to 35% of patients, and stools and gums darken because of bismuth

Prostaglandin analogs such as misoprostol are most effective in the treatment of NSAID-related ulcers. This class of medications has not been approved for use in the United States. Sucralfate is an aluminum hydroxide salt of sucrose octasulfate, a large molecule that acts as a coating agent by possibly enhancing the mucosal barrier. It has been most successful in the treatment of duodenal ulcers. Omeprazole may be used for only 8–12 weeks.

Helicobacter pylori infections may be treated by either double or triple therapy. The use of one regimen over another is related mainly to cost and compliance (Table 14-1).

Referral

Most cases of PUD should respond to initial medical therapy with either antacids or antisecretory drugs within several days to 1 week. If the patient does not respond, referral and consideration of endoscopy should be considered. Individuals with an acute abdomen or unusual pain patterns should be referred to a surgeon. Gallbladder disease may be mistaken for PUD, and vice versa, so consideration should be given to this possibility. Ultrasound may be necessary in cases in which the diagnosis is not clear. Blood in the stool or melanemia should raise suspicion of gastrointestinal cancer in older patients. Individuals over the age of 40 should undergo diagnostic studies of the lower gastrointestinal system in questionable cases. Patients who do not respond may have *H. pylori* infection. Depending on the experience of the physician, referral or consultation should be considered in the evaluation of these patients.

▶ REFERENCES

1. Richter JE, Bradley LA, Castell DO. Esophageal chest pain: current controversies in pathogenesis, diagnosis and therapy. *Ann Intern Med* 1989;110:66–78.

2. Richter JE, Castell DO. Gastroesophageal reflux: pathogenesis, diagnosis, and therapy. *Ann Intern Med* 1982;97:93–103.

3. Harvey RF, Hadley N, Gill TR. Effects of sleeping with the bed-head raised and of ranitidine in patients with severe peptic oesophagitis. *Lancet* 1987;2:1200–3.

4. Soll AH. Pathogenesis of peptic ulcer and implications for therapy. *N Engl J Med* 1990;322:909–16.

5. Peterson WL. Current concepts: *Helicobacter pylori* and peptic ulcer disease. *N Engl J Med* 1991;324:1043–8.

6. Soll AH, Kurata JH, Walsh JH. Ulcer Epidemiology Conference. *Gastroenterology* 1989;96(suppl 2):561–8.

7. Feldman M, Burton ME. Drug therapy: histamine2-receptor antagonists—standard therapy for acid-peptic disease. *N Engl J Med* 1990;323:1672–80,1749–55.

SKIN DISEASE

$\mathbf{A}$ symposium was recently held by the National Institutes of Health on the treatment of androgen excess in women. Their conclusion was that the responsible syndromes represent a continuum and require only a primary care physician, not a gynecologist (for menstrual and ovulatory disorders), a dermatologist (for acne), or an endocrinologist (to rule out congenital adrenal hyperplasia), for treatment. Chapter 15 is a review of acne vulgaris and current treatment options such as antibiotics, mechanical methods, and hormonal manipulations. A common treatment regimen for acne is low-dose contraceptives, local skin care, and broad spectrum antibiotics. None of these approaches requires advanced knowledge or specialty training. Therefore, the treatment of uncomplicated acne may readily be accomplished by a primary care physician. Advanced cases requiring newer medications may require referral.

Chapter 16 reviews skin diseases secondary to solar damage. The incidence of actinar keratosis and melanoma has increased in the past 10 years, especially in the southern United States. A major dilemma for most clinicians is to determine which lesions require biopsy and how the procedure should be performed. Actinar keratosis represents a precursor of other skin malignancies and is easily treated by physical or chemotherapeutic means. Risk determination criteria to identify individuals at high risk for melanoma have become better defined. Prevention is probably the most important aspect of care, and the use of sunblocks and avoidance of sunburns should be stressed. In many cases, a well-performed skin survey is the only management necessary. Suspicious lesions require a biopsy, which is easily performed by the gynecologist, to rule out melanoma.

Acne

$\mathbf{A}$cne, or acne vulgaris, is common reason for a woman to seek medical care; increasingly, women are turning to their primary care provider for treatment rather than a dermatologist.[1] Acne is a self-limited infection that primarily affects adolescents but may be present into the fourth decade.[2] Lesions are heterogeneous and affect the pilosebaceous unit. Keratin from the hair follicle produces acne and its characteristic lesions—pustules, papules, comedones, and nodules—that in advanced cases may lead to pitting and scarring. The goal of therapy is to control the disease to prevent permanent disfigurement.

The predominant lesion is the comedone, which begins in the sebaceous follicle. Keratin formation in affected individuals is altered and in many cases increased. Individuals with acne have certain characteristics, such as large sebaceous glands with increased production of sebum. Free fatty acids (FFAs) are an important component of sebum: if free fatty acids are injected into skin, an inflammatory response follows. Additionally, certain bacteria are essential to acne formation, primarily anaerobic *Propionibacterium acnes* (previously referred to as *Corynebacterium acnes*). These bacteria secrete lipases, chemotactic factors, and proteases and activate complement. However, FFAs and bacteria are not the only factors

193

involved in the production of acne. Linoleic acid, also found in the gland, has an inverse relationship with the severity of the disease. Increasing androgen production at puberty induces sebaceous gland development and increases local conversion of testosterone to dihydrotestosterone at the tissue level. Therapy is directed at altering or eliminating these factors in susceptible individuals.

Diagnosis

Neither history nor laboratory studies are of benefit in diagnosing acne. Physical examination of the face and neck will readily reveal lesions, but the examination should also include the chest, shoulders, and back. Comedones are the primary lesions. They may be open (blackheads) or closed (whiteheads) and accompanied by papules or pustules. Closed comedones may be of greater clinical significance because they are precursors of large inflammatory lesions. Occasionally, folliculitis or rosacea is misdiagnosed as acne.

Treatment

Principles of therapy are directed at altering the local environment of the pilosebaceous unit:

- Correct keratinization patterns of secretion
- Decrease bacteria
- Decrease production of sebum
- Reduce inflammation

Local Therapies.   Facial cleansing has been overemphasized in therapy and should not be stressed as a therapeutic strategy.

Topical agents are usually first-line therapies. Sulfur agents and resorcinol act primarily by drying and pealing the skin but produce erythema and desquamation. Topical vitamin A, formulated as creams and gels, acts primarily as an irritant on comedones. Vitamin A cream in a 0.025% concentration may be used daily without excessive irritation.[3] An important side effect to stress to patients is the enhanced sensitivity to sun, resulting in a sunburn. Benzoyl peroxide preparations are commonly used and available over the counter. The primary actions of benzoyl peroxide are twofold: reduction of bacteria and hydrolysis of triglycerides to FFAs. Dryness and local irritation may limit the usefulness of this medication. Topical antibiotics such as erythromycin (with or without zinc) and clindamycin have been used. Because all the major local therapies work through different mechanisms of action, they may be used in combination without risk of side effects but should not be applied simultaneously.

Physical Therapies. Local extractors ("acne surgery") should not be prescribed because of the difficulty in their use and the potential to inject inflammatory material. Opening closed comedones may be accomplished with a 25-gauge needle, but therapy with topical application of vitamin A is usually more acceptable. Ultraviolet radiation has been used in therapy, but with the heightened awareness of the relationship of radiation with the development of actinar keratosis and malignant melanoma, there is less enthusiasm for this technique. Superficial x-ray therapy was used in the 1960s and 1970s; however, the recognition of a causal relationship with thyroid carcinoma has essentially eliminated the use of this therapy.[4] In severe cases, especially those involving nodular acne, dry ice prepared with acetone may be applied to the face, resulting in a chemical burn; however, healing requires several weeks. Finally, in severe cases, intralesional injection of 0.05–0.25 mL of triamcinolone suspension may be used, which eliminates the need for incision.

Systemic Therapies. Estrogen therapy has a long history in the treatment of acne. Estrogen decreases sebum production and therefore is effective in controlling comedone formation. Originally, 50 μg of ethinyl estradiol was the lowest dose formation thought to be effective, but triphasic formulations have also been found useful.[5] In Europe, estrogen formulations have been combined with cyproterone acetate, a progestational antiandrogen, and found to be effective. The estrogen component of the dose may be lower when used in combination with cyproterone.[6]

Antibiotics, especially the tetracycline derivatives, are successful in the treatment of acne. Their mechanism of action is to decrease FFAs. Several weeks of therapy are required for a response. Initially, 1 gram per day should be given in divided doses. Once control of the condition is gained, the dose can be decreased to 250 mg/day. Other antibiotics have been described as effective including erythromycin, clindamycin, and minocycline. Tetracycline offers the advantage of lower cost and fewer side effects such as the gastrointestinal distress that occurs with erythromycin and the pseudomembranous colitis that accompanies clindamycin use. Tetracycline should not be used if the patient is not using effective contraception because of side effects in the developing fetus. Sulfones (dapsone) have been used in resistant cases, but these medications require monitoring for agranulocytosis and are probably best used by dermatologists.

Isotretinoin is a systemic retinoid that has had significant effects on the treatment of severe persistent acne. Because of the unique side effects of this medication, its use should be reserved for dermatologists. In patients known to use this medication, effective contraception is mandatory.

Referral

Patients with severe disease, especially those with nodular and pitting acne, should be referred because more extensive therapies with various side effects require close monitoring. It is reasonable for obstetrician–gynecologists to use estrogens, systemic antibiotics, and topical therapies to treat acne. Patients with severe acne that involves the back and shoulders should be referred because their conditions are usually difficult to manage and require multiple modes of therapy. Additionally, obstetrician–gynecologists should be cognizant of the side effects of certain medications, such as isotretinoin, and should counsel patients about the use of effective birth control methods, such as oral contraceptives and long-acting injectable progesterones, while they are being treated.

▶ REFERENCES

1. Stern RS, Nelson C. The diminishing role of the dermatologist in the office-based care of cutaneous disease. *J Am Acad Dermatol* 1993;29:773–7.

2. Millikan LE, Shrum JP. An update on common skin diseases. *Postgrad Med* 1992;91:96–102.

3. Strauss JS. Acne vulgaris. In: Fitzpatrick TB, Eisen AZ, Wolff K, Freedberg IM, Austen KF (eds). *Dermatology in general medicine*. New York: McGraw-Hill, 1993;704–24.

4. DeGroot L, Paloyan E. Thyroid carcinoma and radiation. A Chicago endemic. *JAMA* 1975;225:487–91.

5. Anderson FD. Selectivity and minimal androgenicity of norgestimate in monophasic and triphasic oral contraceptives. *Acta Obstet Gynecol Scand Suppl* 1992;156:15–21.

6. Colver GB, Mortimer PS, Dawber RPR. Cyproterone acetate and two doses of oestrogen in female acne: a double blind comparison. *Br J Dermatol* 1988;118:95–9.

CHAPTER 16

Actinar Keratosis and Malignant Melanoma

In the Caucasian population, malignant melanoma has been increasing for decades at a rate of 4–8% per year. It currently is the fasting growing cancer in the United States,[1] with an estimated 32,000 new cases in 1991. Melanoma has surpassed malignancies of the brain, larynx, trachea, and thyroid in frequency and is approaching that of colorectal carcinoma. Fortunately, survival is also increasing, and the prognosis is better in women than in men.

Actinar keratosis (AK or solar keratosis) is a precancerous lesion of the skin that is related to sun exposure and is associated with squamous cell carcinoma of the skin and malignant melanoma. Currently, a major effort is underway to educate the public about the hazards of solar and ultraviolet radiation and sun exposure. Many dermatologists and epidemiologists feel that a strong link exists between sun exposure and the development of these lesions.

► ACTINAR KERATOSIS

History

Actinar keratosis is most commonly found in older, blue-eyed individuals who are prone to freckling. In sunny areas, it may be found in teenagers and young adults and increases in incidence with age.[2] Additional risk factors are immunocompromised conditions, such as those that occur in transplant patients. To further support the link between solar radiation and AK, it has been shown that reducing sun exposure in childhood may result in a reduced occurrence of squamous cell carcinoma with aging. There is a fivefold increase in malignant melanoma in patients with AK.

Diagnosis

Actinar keratosis typically occurs on sun-exposed body regions in middle-aged to older individuals. Lesions range in color from skin color to red-brown to yellowish-black macules or papules with a dry adherent scale. In many cases, the palpable granular-feeling lesions may be recognized better by feel than by appearance. Solar elastosis (lack of cutaneous support from sun-damaged skin) may be associated with the formation of AK. In many cases, lesions are multiple rather than solitary and are mildly tender.

Spreading pigmented actinar keratosis is a variant commonly found on the face. The lesion is greater than 1 cm in size, displays varying degrees of pigmentation, and spreads in a centrifugal fashion. Other variants are the large, projectile line mass referred to as a cutaneous horn. Lesions that are indurated, erythematous, and increasing in diameter with erosions are suspicious for squamous cell carcinoma and should be biopsied. If the diagnosis is questionable but the lesions are difficult of identify, topical application of 5-fluorouracil will induce erythema.

Actinar keratosis is usually fairly easy to diagnose. Differential diagnosis is seborrheic keratosis (distinguished by pits and furrows under a magnifying glass) and melanocytic nevi. When in doubt, biopsy! The definitive test to perform, especially when confronted by dermatologic lesions, is either an excision skin biopsy, which is preferable, or punch biopsy. If punch biopsy is chosen for cosmetic reasons, the thickest and most abnormally appearing area should be selected.

Treatment

Prevention by avoidance of ultraviolet radiation is the best treatment; unfortunately, in most cases preventive therapy occurs decades too late. However, women with children at high risk should be reminded of the correlation between sun damage and lesions. Suspicious lesions should be biopsied before initiating therapy. The most useful therapy is cryosurgery with liquid nitrogen for isolated lesions. Larger areas should be treated with topical 5% 5-fluorouracil cream. The cream should be applied daily for 2–4 weeks. Erythema and exfoliation should follow and a therapeutic response may take up to 2 months to occur after completion of therapy. Fortunately, only 12–13% of patients progress to carcinoma, and squamous cell carcinoma is not locally aggressive and has virtually no metastatic potential.

Referral

Most of these lesions may easily be cared for in the office with minimal investment of equipment. Referral is indicated if the practitioner does not desire to care for these patients. Facial lesions should be considered for referral to a dermatologist for cosmetic considerations.

▶ MALIGNANT MELANOMA

As the incidence of malignant melanoma has grown over the past five decades, so too has awareness of the disorder on the part of primary care physicians. There are four different varieties of malignant melanoma: (1) superficial spreading melanoma, which is the most common and will be the subject of this discussion; (2) lentigo maligna melanoma, which is the least common but has the strongest link to sun exposure and damage; (3) nodular melanoma, which is rare and not sunlight dependent; and (4) acral-lentiginous melanoma, which is common in African–Americans and Asians and occurs primarily on the palms of the hands and soles of the feet.

History

The etiology of the increased incidence of malignant melanoma is probably multifactoral and includes a shift in demographics to more people living in the sun belt and increase in leisure time for outdoor activities. Known risk factors for the development of malignant melanoma are:

- Blond or red hair with fair skin
- Blue eyes
- Tendency to sunburn or freckling, frequency and intensity of sunburns
- Inability to tan (skin phototype I [i.e., skin phototype III tans easily])
- Upper socioeconomic status
- Family history of melanoma (6–12%) or history of non-melanoma skin cancer

- Melanocytic nevi with increased numbers of nevi, large nevi, and nevi of variegated color with an irregular border
- Congenital or dysplastic nevi

Individuals with these risk factors should be counseled concerning their risk and possible preventative behaviors such as avoidance of sunlight and the use of sun blocks when exposure to sunlight is unavoidable. The increase in incidence is primarily found in men more than women and on certain areas of the body. Episodic areas of exposure, such as the trunk (found more commonly in men) and the legs (more commonly found in women), have increased dramatically over the past several decades. Additionally, a shift in age distribution has been apparent with the site: trunk and leg malignant melanoma occurs most commonly between the ages of 40 and 60, whereas malignant melanoma of the head increases after age 50.[3] Finally, age of sun overexposure and damage is important: individuals are less susceptible if the damage occurred prior to age 9 and after age 40.[4]

The history should include how long the lesion has been present, growth characteristics, change in color or border, and recent bleeding or ulceration. It should also include information about sun exposure and family history.

Diagnosis

Physical examination of the entire body should be performed. This may be performed in segments so the patient is not forced to be totally disrobed. Side lighting should be used with a hand-held lens, and inspection with a Wood's light should be performed. The location and size of any suspicious-looking lesions should be documented. If the lesions are very suspicious looking, biopsy should be performed. Evidence of lymphadenopathy and hepatosplenomegaly should be determined, and any abnormal symptoms should be evaluated. Chest x-ray and complete blood count are the only ancillary studies necessary. Pregnancy was once considered a high-risk group for poor outcome, but recent data do not support this contention.[5] Authorities do recommend, however, that pregnancy be avoided for 2 years after diagnosis if the lesion is >1.5 mm in thickness.[6] Because most malignant melanomas of the female genital tract are found on the vulva, the obstetrician–gynecologist should primarily biopsy these lesions.

Any suspicious lesion should be biopsied. The presence of five cardinal features constitute criteria to biopsy: symmetry, irregular and scalloped border, mottled appearance, large diameter, and elevation with surface distortion. A full elliptical biopsy should be performed with adequate depth to reach the fat layer.

Tumorigenesis and staging are important in understanding the growth and hence prognosis of malignant melanoma. There are three stages of malignant melanoma.

- Stage I: Localized disease with no palpable regional lymph nodes (most common sites of lymph node metastases are ilioinguinal, axillary, intraparotid, and cervical lymph nodes). There is no histologic evidence of tumor in the regional lymph nodes.
- Stage II: Palpable regional lymph nodes with histological evidence of melanoma in regional lymph nodes.
- Stage III: Presence of distant metastases with histopathologic documentation.

Tumor initiation usually begins superficially and then invades progressively. Stages of tumor in formation are:

- Benign melanocytic nevi
- Melanocytic nevi with architectural and cytologic atypia
- Primary malignant melanoma, radial growth phase
- Primary malignant melanoma, vertical growth phase
- Metastatic malignant melanoma

The transition from stage 3 or the radial growth phase to stage 4 or vertical growth phase is probably the most important prognostic factor. Similar to squamous cell carcinoma of the cervix, as tumor depth of invasion increases, so does the potential for the cancer to enter vascular and lymphatic spaces and, therefore, for distant metastasis to occur. This has led to two primary classification schemes: the Breslow thickness based on anatomic levels of invasion and the Clark anatomic level of invasion. The Breslow system measures from the granular cell layer (top layer of squamous epithelium) of the epidermis to the greatest depth of invasion using an ocular micrometer. In Stage I disease, the Breslow system has proved to be the single most important prognosticator of disease.[7] Clark levels are based on five anatomical levels: I = intraepidermal, II = in papillary dermis, III = fills papillary dermis, IV = reticular dermis, and V = enters fat. A primary problem with this system is deciding where to discriminate in defining levels.

There are other variables important in prognosis of Stage I malignant melanoma. Women have a more favorable prognosis than men, mostly because of the prevalence of lower extremity lesions, which on average are thinner. Additionally, women have better survival rates, even when the vertical stage of tumor growth has been reached.[8] Older age has been associated with increased tumor thickness and hence poor prognosis. Level of tumor progression, histogenic type, and degree of tumor ulceration are also important factors in prognosis.

Referral

Once malignant melanoma has been diagnosed, referral to an oncologic general surgeon should be initiated. Controversy exists regarding the width of incisions and whether regional lymph nodes should undergo dissection or biopsy. Malignant melanoma is primarily a surgical disease and at present no adjuvant therapy such as chemotherapy and/or immunotherapy has been found effective. Additionally, if a patient has a history of melanoma or dysplastic nevi syndrome, close follow-up by a dermatologist is probably indicated. As with actinar keratosis, facial lesions should be considered for referral to a dermatologist for cosmetic considerations.

▶ REFERENCES

1. Boring CC, Squires TS, Tong T. Cancer statistics, 1991. CA *Cancer J Clin* 1991;41:19–36.

2. Marks R. Solar keratoses. *Br J Dermatol* 1990;122(suppl 35):49–54.

3. Holman CDJ, Armstrong BK. Pigmentary traits, ethnic origin, benign nevi, and family history of risk factors for cutaneous malignant melanoma. *J Natl Cancer Inst* 1984;72:257–66.

4. Holly EA, Aston DA, Cress RD, Ahn DK, Kristiansen JJ. Cutaneous melanoma in women. I. Exposure to sunlight, ability to tan, and other risk factors related to ultraviolet light. *Am J Epidemiol* 1995;141(10):923–33.

5. Reintgen DS, McCarthy Jr KS, Vollmer R, Cox E, Seigler HF. Malignant melanoma and pregnancy. *Cancer* 1985;55:1340–4.

6. Clark WH Jr, Elder DE, Guerry D IV, et al. Model predicting survival in Stage I melanoma based on tumor progression. *J Natl Cancer Inst* 1989;81:1893–1904.

7. Breslow A. Tumor thickness, level of invasion, and node dissection in Stage I cutaneous melanoma. *Ann Surg* 1975;182:572–75.

8. Clark WH Jr, Elder DE, Guerry D IV, et al. Model predicting survival in Stage I melanoma based on tumor progression. *J Natl Cancer Inst* 1989;81:1893–1904.

NEUROPSYCHIATRY

Chapter 17 is devoted to depression, probably the
most common psychiatric syndrome and an often unrecognized cause of physician visits. Unfortunately, most
Americans perceive psychiatric disorders as a sign of
individual weakness and not as true "diseases." Despite
this bias, depressive illnesses cost the United States bil-
lions of dollars a year and they remain underrecognized
in most physician's offices, even when patients have obvious vegetative symptoms and signs. The introduction
of selective serotonin reuptake inhibitor (SSRI) antidepressants has been a boom to patients and practitioners
because of their low side-effect profiles. Questions, however, are surfacing concerning the appropriateness of
their use in some cases.

Chapter 18 is a review of headache disorders and
newer therapeutic options. Headaches are a source of
annoyance common to most people. The practitioner, despite the ubiquitous nature of cephalgia, should obtain a
thorough history to distinguish between the different
types of headache. Most women have tension and migraine syndromes and rarely are affected by cluster head-

aches. Many patients complain of "migraine" headaches purely because recent tension headaches seem worse. Close examination, however, will reveal the lack of classic symptoms, such as characteristic aura. Newer medications have been extremely helpful in relieving migraine syndromes. Additionally, commonly used antihypertensive agents have also been found useful in many individuals.

CHAPTER 17

Depression

Depression is a common problem that is probably under-recognized by most practitioners. The incidence has increased every decade since 1900. As women are confronted with societal pressures and influences, they too have experienced an increase in stress from balancing home and the work place, contributing to depression. Women have a lifetime risk of 15–25% and are twice as likely as men to suffer from depression. This statistic may be misleading, however; women are also more likely than men to seek care.[1] Despite the relative high frequency of depression, however, less than 25% of patients receive treatment.[2] The reason for this is twofold: patients feel that it is a sign of weakness or illness to ask for help and symptoms are viewed by doctors as "normal" or expected reactions to stress. Physical symptoms are more acceptable than emotional symptoms, which may explain the prevalence of chronic pelvic pain versus depression.

History

The etiology of depression has not been well-established and different theories have been advanced. Depression has long been studied to identify underlying endogenous biochemical and biological factors. The results of many studies have shown the presence of abnormal regulation of norepinephrine and decreased serotonin activity accompanying depression. Knowledge of these changes has been useful in pharmaceutical research and development of newer medications such as selective serotonin reuptake inhibitors (SSRIs). Psychological factors, such as unexpressed anger, unresolved grief, and learned helplessness, have been considered operative in behavioral theories.

Even though depression is considered to have an endogenous component, there are external pressures that may precipitate a major depressive disorder. Although these episodes are thought to be "situational" disorders or depression, they may herald the beginning of a major episode. In women, specific conditions may be more likely to initiate an episode: (1) early childhood loss or prolonged illness of a parent; (2) domestic violence, physical and sexual abuse; (3) genetic predisposition; (4) socioeconomic deprivation; and (5) life-style stress, especially that of multiple roles (worker, mother, and spouse).[2]

Women are more susceptible to depression at certain times in their lives. The health care provider for women should be attuned to these events and the accompanying risk of depression. Perinatal loss has been underemphasized as a time of grief, anger, and associated depression. Support for the patient and her family should be provided at 6-week, 3-month, and 6-month intervals. Infertility is another recognized cause of depression in reproductive age women. Group therapy may be useful for these individuals. Pregnancy, particularly during the postpartum period, is well-known as a time for major depression. Many patients with postpartum depression have a history of previous depression and should be monitored closely. Finally, old age and the menopause are times of physiologic and psychological changes. The concept of involutional melancholia should be discarded, and specific etiologies in the social and psychological context pursued.[3]

Once an individual has experienced a major depressive episode, the likelihood of additional episodes increases. Therefore, it is important in the initial history to obtain information on previous episodes and their courses. Attempts should be made to classify the episodes, specifically in relation to psychotic behavior and suicidal ideation, gestures, and attempts. Patients with severe episodes may require hospitalization and intensive pharmacologic and psychological support.

Information about the completeness of past remissions should be sought. If patterns of depression are episodic and of short duration, simple office counseling and follow-up will suffice. Additionally, previous treatments for depression, including medication type and dosage, should be documented. Any history of manic episodes is important and, if present, will probably dictate referral. Mania has been described in up to 30% of patients with depression. Historically, these patients have a history of higher activity levels, increased energy, pressured speech, decreased need for sleep, and self-overestimation of abilities. In many depression sufferers, a history of hypomania may be obtained. Hypomania is similar to mania, but without the psychotic episodes or fugue states.

Substance abuse, as a method of self-medication, is more common among those with depression. Patients with a long history of depression who present with acute symptoms may be noncompliant with prescribed medication. These individuals "don't like drugs" and can "handle it themselves."

Diagnosis

It is normal to experience depressive symptoms for short periods in response to loss, disappointment, or change. True depression, however, extends beyond feeling sadness and becomes a dominant affect or *mood disorder*. The disorder is characterized by changes in mood, thinking, and behavior and by biological alterations:

- *Mood (Emotional Tone).* lack of motivation, apathy, sadness, tearfulness, unhappiness, discouragement, and hostility. The first clue to an underlying depression may be *anhedonia,* or the loss of capacity to feel happiness.
- *Negative Thinking.* self-blame, worthlessness, guilt, and a generalized feeling that things cannot get better. Recurrent thoughts of dying, suicidal ideation, or suicide attempts are specific warning signs.
- *Cognitive Disorders.* slow thinking, difficulty remembering, indecisiveness, and inability to concentrate.
- *Behavior Changes.* passiveness, dependency, and helplessness. These behaviors may manifest in marital discord, alienation of friends, problems at work, and self-destructive behavior (e.g., accident proneness).
- *Biologic Functions.* sleep disturbance and eating disorders. Many patients have trouble falling and staying asleep, whereas some will sleep too much. Appetite and weight can be increased or decreased, and "energy levels" are typically decreased. Examples of other physical problems may be "weakness," fatigue, dizziness, and constipation.

Depression has been classified into different clinical types to standardize research, communication, and evaluation of therapies. These classifications, currently outlined in the fourth edition of the *Diagnostic and Statistical Manual of Mental Disorders,* or DSM-IV™, are updated regularly.[4] Following are important classifications to recognize in primary care:

- Major change of mood: the loss of ability to experience pleasure.
- Major depression characterized by an endogenous, melancholic, or vegetative state.
- Major depression with psychosis: these patients may have delusions, loss of reality testing, and hallucinations.
- Dysthymia: a chronic, low-grade depressive episode that lasts for at least 2 years.
- Bipolar personality disorder, previously called the manic–depressive disorder.
- Seasonal affective disorder (SAD): light-related; increased incidence in fall/winter when days are shorter.

In most cases, episodes first occur during the reproductive ages, but depression may begin at any age. Additionally, if an individual has one single major depressive episode, the risk of a second episode is 50–60%. Of particular significance and concern is the 15% chance of suicide associated with a major depressive episode.

The natural history of acute depression is for many patients to have several recurrences. Bipolar depression recurs twice as often as unipolar depression. Unfortunately, each recurrence lasts longer and is usually more severe. In 50% of patients with acute depression, symptoms remit spontaneously. In the remaining patients, symptoms will improve with prolonged therapy in 35%, but up to 15% of patients remain ill.

There is no laboratory test available to aid in the diagnosis of depression. However, depression may affect the results of other tests. This phenomenon of altered test results is alluded to as proof of the organic nature of depression. The results of the following studies are affected by depression.

- Dexamethasone suppression test. Up to 50% of depressed patients will fail to suppress endogenous cortisol after the short or single-dose test (1 mg of dexamethasone given at bedtime with an 8 am cortisol sample drawn).
- Thyrotropin-releasing hormone (TRH) stimulation test. One-third of patients will have a blunted rise in thyroid-stimulating hormone levels after a 500-µg injection of TRH.
- A sleep electroencephalogram (EEG) will reveal that 80% of patients with depression have decreased rapid eye movement (REM).

Depression may be the manifestation of other underlying diseases and a differential diagnosis should be considered.[5] Even though depression is usually endogenous in many younger patients, the following other illness should be considered:

- Viral infections, specifically hepatitis and mononucleosis
- Cancer, especially pancreatic cancer in the elderly
- Collagen vascular diseases
- Endocrine disorders, including hypothyroidism, hypo-adrenalism (Addison's disease), and panhypopituitarism
- Stroke in the elderly, especially if coexisting hypertension and peripheral vascular disease are present
- Organic brain disease including dementia and Alzheimer's disease

Eating disorders and substance abuse may cause major depression.[6] Certain gynecologic conditions are commonly associated with underlying or unrecognized depression. These ailments can also be among the most challenging conditions to diagnose and treat. Common gynecologic conditions related to depression include chronic pelvic pain, idiopathic vulvodynia, vaginal pain and burning, poorly characterized dyspareunia, and incapacitating and severe premenstrual symptoms. Exaggerated or prolonged depression can also be associated with hysterectomy, infertility, mastectomy, and menopause.

Certain medicines are known to produce depression in susceptible individuals and may be dose related. Commonly prescribed medications that may produce depression include:

- Oral contraceptives, usually related to a specific progesterone
- Propranolol
- Bromocriptine
- Cimetidine, usually in the elderly and may cause confusion
- Digitalis
- Phenytoin
- Spironolactone
- Reserpine
- Withdrawal syndromes with amphetamine, cocaine, and sedatives/tranquilizers
- Alcohol

Treatment

Treatment should initially focus on resolution of immediate problems such as suicide risk; then it should be directed to long-term therapy such as medication and counseling. Electroconvulsive therapy is used in refractory depression and is outside the scope of the primary care physician. Most individuals who resort to suicide visit their primary care physician shortly before death. In the initial assessment of the depressed patient, the patient should be asked about suicidal thoughts and ideation. If these feelings are present, evaluation of the possibility and immediacy of a suicide attempt or gesture should be considered and documented. Most gynecologists develop a third sense about their patients. Use it! If the patient seems overburdened, with poor eye contact and shutting out all suggestions, consider the possibility of suicide! If the possibility of suicide is real, plans for hospitalization and immediate transfer should be implemented. Patients at high risk should be placed under close observation until the risk diminishes.

Psychotherapy appears to be as effective as pharmacotherapy in the treatment of mild to moderate depression.[6] Principles of psychotherapy require that problems are openly discussed and then resolved through insight, emotional support, and an understanding gained from the patient–therapist relationship. Most problems in women evolve from a negative viewpoint of themselves and their expanded role in the workplace, home, and society.[4] As the number of single-parent households increases, the burden on the responsible adult to maintain a home will only increase. Psychotherapy should be directed at positive thinking, realistic appraisal of self-worth, and enhancement of independence and autonomy. Unfortunately, psychotherapy requires certain time commitments, which may be limited in the busy gynecologic practice.

The development of new classes of medications for depression has revolutionized treatment. Medication was originally considered only for patients with severe depression. In current practice, however, mild to moderate depression is treated with newer drugs that have less distressing side effects. The major classes of medications are tricyclics, heterocyclics, selective serotonin reuptake inhibitors (SSRIs), and monoamine oxidase (MAO) inhibitors. Monamine oxidase inhibitors have multiple serious side effects and require close monitoring. Unless the gynecologist uses this class of drugs frequently, they are probably outside the scope of usual practice and therefore will not be discussed.

Tricyclics were the original antidepressant medications available. Major formulations in this class include amitriptyline, desipramine, doxepin, imipramine, and nortriptyline. Side effects common to most of these drugs include anticholinergic effects such as dry mouth, blurred vision, urinary hesitancy, and constipation. Imipramine is probably used more for its side effect of increasing urethral tone and relaxing the detrusor, as a result of its alpha-adrenergic-stimulating properties, than as an antidepressant. Many patients feel drowsy or "hung-over" when using tricyclics. Other distressing side effects include orthostatic hypotension, cardiac arrhythmia, and, in some cases, weight gain. Because of the long half-lives and renal excretion of these medications, dosages should be closely monitored in the elderly. In most cases, these drugs are given in a single evening dose and require up to 3 weeks for therapeutic efficacy. Finally, these drugs may be lethal used in combination with MAO inhibitors.

Common agents and dosage ranges are:

Amitriptyline (Elavil, Endep)	75–300 mg hs
Desipramine (Norpramin, Pertofrane)	75–300 mg hs
Doxepin (Adapin, Sinequan)	75–300 mg hs
Imipramine (Janimine, Tofranil)	75–300 mg hs
Nortriptyline (Aventyl, Pamelor)	40–200 mg hs

The heterocyclics were the next class of medications introduced for the treatment of depression. Examples of this group of medications include amoxapine, bupropion, maprotiline, and trazodone. The major advantages over the tricyclics were the lessening of anticholinergic side effects, orthostatic hypotension, and cardiac arrhythmias. Drowsiness is decreased but still present. As a group they require a once-daily dosage and may be lethal used in combination with MAO inhibitors. The usual response is delayed and may require up to 4–6 weeks for an effect.

Common agents and dosage ranges are:

Amoxapine (Asendin)	10–40 mg hs
Bupropion (Wellbutrin)	225–450 mg hs
Maprotiline (Ludiomil)	100–225 mg hs
Trazodone (Desyrel)	150–600 mg hs

The newest agents available that have dramatically changed therapy in depression are the SSRIs. Medications in this class are fluoxetine, paroxetine, and sertraline. These medications have virtually no anticholinergic side effects or drowsiness. Cardiovascular side effects are also essentially eliminated. Gastrointestinal distress, however, is more prevalent with this class of medication. Because of the absence of side effects, these medications have exploded in popularity in the past decade. Effects may not be noted for 4–8 weeks, and use with MAO inhibitors may cause fatal side effects. Questions about their widespread use has been raised, even in the popular press.

Common agents and dosage ranges are:

Fluoxetine (Prozac)	10–40 mg hs
Paroxetine (Paxil)	20–50 mg hs
Sertraline (Zoloft)	50–150 mg hs

The effects of these medications are (1) to decrease the lack of appetite and weight loss, (2) to increase energy, (3) to decrease suicidal thoughts, and (4) to decrease negative thoughts such as helplessness, excessive guilt, and hopelessness. Unfortunately, they may decrease a sense of pleasure derived from activities.

In general, medication should be used for 4 weeks to 6 months. When clinical response has been reached, the medication should be withdrawn slowly. The effects of medication alone, however, are limited if environmental and personal behaviors are unchanged. Medication should never be used solely to treat depression without ongoing counseling and behavioral therapy.

Special situations include the elderly, treatment of bipolar disorders, and seasonal affective disorders (SADs). Elderly patients may respond to stimulants (e.g., dextroamphetamine). Patients with bipolar disorders, especially those with mania, will need treatment and prophylaxis with lithium. Finally, for individuals with SAD, bright-light therapy, frequent walks during the day, and a well-planned vacation may be helpful.

Referral

Patients with a history of major depressive episodes lasting greater than 4–6 months should be considered for referral. These patients may require multiple medications and intensive cide gestures and attempts are probably best treated by a psychiatrist. A history of prior psychotic behavior, manic fugue states, and severe eating disorders will also be best served by a psychiatrist. If initial attempts with single medications such as tricyclics, heterocyclics, and SSRIs are unsuccessful, referral should strongly be considered. Finally, if the physician either does not communicate well with the patient, or the patient does not respond to the physician's efforts, timely referral is the best route for all parties.

► REFERENCES

1. Notman MT. Depression in women. Psychoanalytical concepts. *Psychiatr Clin North Am* 1989;12:221–30.

2. McGrath E, Ketia GP, Strickland BR, Russo NF. Women and depression: risk factors and treatment issues. Washington DC: American Psychological Association, 1990.

3. ACOG Technical Bulletin #182, *Depression in women,* July 1993.

4. *Diagnostic and Statistical Manual of Mental Disorders.* DSM-IV™. Washington DC: American Psychiatric Association, 1994.

5. Rodin G, Voshart K. Depression in the medically ill, an overview. *Am J Psychiatry* 1986;143:696–705.

6. Depression Guideline Panel. *Depression in primary care: detection, diagnosis, and treatment,* No. 5. Rockville MD: US Department of Health and Human Services, Public Health Service, Agency for Health Care Policy and Research, 1993. AHCPR publication #93-0552.

► CHAPTER **18**

Headache

Headache is a complaint that affects almost 99% of women during their lifetime. Headache is usually part of a primary headache disorder. In some cases, headache may be an associated symptom of another illness such as a brain tumor, cerebral hemorrhage, or meningitis. In 1988, the International Headache Society (IHS) published criteria for classification and diagnosis of a broad range of headache disorders.[1]

Classification of headaches is important in prescribing therapy. The most common headaches described are tension-type headaches (TTHs), both episodic and chronic tension headaches, and migraine headaches with and without aura. Cluster headaches are uncommon in women but have classic symptoms that are easily recognizable.

Tension-Type Headaches. With TTHs, pain is typically described as bilateral; dull, deep, or bandlike; mild to moderate in severity; not aggravated by exertion; and lasting from 30 minutes to 7 days. Patients with episodic tension-type headaches (ETTHs) should be distinguished from those with chronic tension-type headaches (CTTHs). Both have similar symptoms; however, ETTHs occur <15 days a month, whereas patients with CTTHs have symptoms >15 days/month and usually daily. Many patients with CTTH overuse medications,

223

including over-the-counter headache remedies. As a group, these patients will rarely give an accurate history of medication use and may suffer from depression.[2] It may be difficult to differentiate TTH from migraine without aura because both may be episodic, bilateral, nonthrobbing, and of moderate severity, with associated anorexia, photophobia, and phonophobia. Gastrointestinal symptoms are more common with migraine syndromes and rarely seen with TTH. Following are characteristics of ETTH:

- Headache lasting from 30 minutes to 7 days
- At least two of the following pain characteristics:
  (a) Pressing/tightening (nonpulsating) quality
  (b) Mild or moderate intensity (may inhibit but does not prohibit activities)
- Bilateral location
- No aggravation by routine physical activity
- Both of the following symptoms:
  (a) No nausea or vomiting (anorexia may occur)
  (b) Photophobia and phonophobia are absent, or one but not the other is present
- At least 10 previous headache episodes with number of headache days <180/year or <15/month

Migraine. Migraine syndrome is an episodic headache disorder usually lasting 4–24 hours, commonly initiated by a prodromal phase and preceded by an aura. Most sufferers have their initial migraine headache in childhood or early adulthood (women are more susceptible than men in adulthood). The headache, of moderate to severe intensity, may be unilateral or bilateral and is described as throbbing. Attacks are associated with photophobia, lightheadedness with nausea, and sensitivity to movement. The menstrual cycle may contribute to migraine attacks.[3] Once the attack begins, the individual retreats to a dark room and attempts to sleep. Migraines are classified by the presence of aura (classic migraine) or without aura (common migraine). Diagnostic criteria for common migraine are as follows:[1]

- Headache lasting from 4 to 72 hours
- Headache has at least two of the following characteristics:
  - (a) Unilateral location
  - (b) Pulsating quality
  - (c) Moderate or severe intensity
  - (d) Aggravation by routine physical activity
- During headache at least one of the following:
  - (a) Nausea and/or vomiting
  - (b) Photophobia and phonophobia
- At least five attacks have occurred fulfilling the above criteria

Classic migraines are described as having an "aura" (complex of focal neurological symptoms) preceding an attack. Following are the types of auras described:

- Homonymous visual disturbance, bright scintillating lights in a zigzag pattern moving across the field of vision, sparks or flashing lights, and visual illusions or distortions
- Unilateral weakness, paresthesias and/or numbness
- Aphasia or unclassifiable speech difficulty

Following are criteria for the diagnosis of migraine with aura (classic migraine):[1]

- At least three of the following four characteristics are present:
  - (a) One or more fully reversible aura symptoms indicating focal cerebral cortical or brain stem dysfunction
  - (b) At least one aura symptom develops gradually over more than 4 minutes or two or more symptoms occur in succession
  - (c) No aura symptom lasts more than 60 minutes
  - (d) Headache follows aura with a free interval of less than 60 minutes (it may also begin before or simultaneously with the aura)
- At least two attacks have occurred fulfilling the aforementioned criteria

Status migrainosus refers to bouts of migraine that last longer than 72 hours and may be associated with nausea, vomiting, and dehydration.

Cluster Headache. Cluster headache is a nonfamilial disorder predominantly affecting men. Attacks are brief (30–90 minutes), usually occur in clusters lasting weeks, and are described as excruciatingly severe. When they occur, they are frequent (hence "cluster") and associated with unilateral autonomic signs, such as tearing and a runny nose. Prodrome, aura, postdrome, and associated gastrointestinal symptoms are absent.

Diagnosis

History is the most important tool in diagnosis since most headache patients have normal neurologic and physical examinations. The following factors should be considered in the evaluation:

- Present illness: new, progressive, or recurrent headache
- Age at onset
- Location
- Frequency
- Onset, duration, character, and severity: migraine is throbbing; cluster is deep and boring; tension-type headache is dull and bandlike
- Course: a progressively worsening headache is worrisome
- Presence of prodromes and aura
- Associated signs and symptoms: nasal congestion, tearing (cluster); nausea and vomiting (migraine); teeth grinding and neck tenderness (TTH)
- Signs of depression and cognitive dysfunction
- Signs of neurologic dysfunction: weakness, paresthesia, aphasia, diplopia, visual loss, vertigo, and faintness
- Precipitating factors: bright light, fatigue, loss of sleep, hypoglycemia, stress, certain drugs, alcohol, food additives, and menstruation can provoke migraine
- Family history
- Multiplicity: patients frequently have different headache types and do not suffer from one particular pattern

The physical and neurologic examinations can rule out systemic and neurologic causes of headache. Laboratory testing can exclude secondary causes of headache, provide a baseline for potential side effects, monitor drug levels, and confirm or exclude medication overuse. Some patients will require neurodiagnostic testing or a lumbar puncture or both to rule out an organic central nervous system cause of headache.

Patients may have headaches that could signal a more severe problem. Following are causes for concern that warrant further evaluation:

- The "first or worst headache" of the patient's life (particularly if it is of acute onset)
- Progressively worsening headache
- A headache associated with fever, nausea, and vomiting that cannot be explained by a systemic illness
- A headache associated with focal neurologic findings, papilledema, a stiff neck, or changes in consciousness or in cognition (such as difficulty in reading, writing, or thinking)
- No obvious identifiable headache etiology
- Medication overuse
- Failure to respond to therapy

If any of these conditions exist, medical or neurologic consultation, imaging studies (magnetic resonance imaging or computed tomography scanning), or lumbar puncture may be indicated.

The first or worst headache of a patient's life should be assumed to be an acute neurologic disorder. If the current headache is similar to multiple prior headaches, there is less risk of a new problem.

Acute recurrent headaches are usually TTH or migraine; subarachnoid hemorrhage, cerebrovascular insufficiency, intermittent hydrocephalus, pheochromocytoma, trigeminal neuralgia, cluster headache, and pseudotumor cerebri are less common causes. Subacute headache, present for days or weeks, may be the beginning of CTTH but usually signifies a primary neurologic disorder and demands a complete neurologic evaluation. Chronic daily headache may be related to analgesic overuse, pseudotumor cerebri, or an underlying psychological problem. Patients may present to the emergency department with the "last straw" syndrome. The patients typically have CTTH with superimposed, more severe migraine headache.

Headache should be evaluated with the same intensity and completeness as any other clinical condition. Migraine headache should be diagnosed only after other conditions that can mimic it have been excluded. Diagnostic testing cannot replace, but should be an adjunct to, a comprehensive history and physical examination.

Treatment

Prophylactic treatment is designed to reduce the frequency and severity of headache attacks.[4] Abortive treatment is aimed at stopping individual attacks, reducing the severity and duration of head pain, and alleviating associated symptoms, including nausea and vomiting. Patients can use abortive headache medication even if they are using prophylactic agents. Abortive headache medications include analgesics, anxiolytics, nonsteroidal anti-inflammatory drugs (NSAIDs), ergotamine, steroids, major tranquilizers, narcotics, and, most recently, sumatriptan, a direct-acting serotonin agonist (Table 18-1).

Prophylactic medication use should be considered when (1) a patient has at least two or three attacks per month; (2) the attacks are incapacitating, associated with focal neurologic signs, or of prolonged duration; (3) the patient is unable to

▶ TABLE 18-1 Abortive Medications

Simple Analgesics = Caffeine

• Acetaminophen 250 mg and/or aspirin 250 mg, caffeine 65 mg PO. Limit dose to 1 g stat, 4 g/day. Avoid daily use (renal insufficiency).

Combination Analgesics = Butalbital

• Aspirin 325 mg or acetaminophen 325 mg, butalbital 50 mg, caffeine 40 mg PO. Limit dose to 1 or 2 tablets stat, 6 tablets/attack, and 24 tablets month.

• Aspirin 650 mg or acetaminophen 325 mg; butalbital 50 mg PO.

Combination Analgesics with Narcotics

• Aspirin 325 mg, butalbital 50 mg, caffeine 40 mg, codeine phosphate 30 mg PO. Limit dose to 1 or 2 stat, 6 tablets/attack, and 16/month.

• Aspirin 325 mg, codeine 30 mg PO.

• Acetaminophen 125, 300, or 325 mg; codeine 7.5, 15, 30, or 60 mg PO.

Nonsteroidal Anti-inflammatory Drugs (MID = maximum initial dose)

• Naproxen sodium 275 mg PO: MID 825 mg. Up to maximum dose may be taken stat.

• Ibuprofen 200, 300, 400, 600, or 800 mg PO: MID 800 mg.

• Meclofenamate sodium 50 or 100 mg PO: MID 100 mg.

• Indomethacin 25, 50, or 75 mg PO: MID 50 mg.

• Ketoprofen 25, 50, or 75 mg PO: MID 75 mg.

• Diclofenac sodium 25, 50, or 75 mg PO: MID 75 mg.

Sympathomimetic Agents

• Isometheptene, acetaminophen, dichloralphenazone (Isocom, Midrin) PO. Dose: 2 tablets stat, can repeat in 1 hour (limit: 3 times/week).

Ergotamine Tartrate

• Caffeine 100 mg, ergotamine tarttrate 1 mg PO/PR. Dose: up to 6 mg (oral) or 2 suppositories stat. Limit monthly use to 8 events or 24 mg (oral) or to 12 suppositories.[a]

continued

► **TABLE 18-1   Continued**

Dihydroergotamine Mesylate

• Dihydroergotamine mesylate 1 mg/mL, ampule IM or IV. Dose: up to 1 mg stat, 3 mg/day. Limit monthly use to 12 events or 18 ampules.

Serotonin Agonists

• Sumatriptan SC 6 mg; can be repeated after 1 hour. (Limit: 2 injections/24hr).

[a]Keep 3 days between dosing with ergotamine in patients with frequent or daily headache.

cope with his or her headache; and (4) there are contraindications or adverse reactions to abortive medication. Following are guidelines for the use of prophylactic medication:

• Ensure that the patient is not taking medications that would interfere with therapy and is not overusing abortive medications.
• Be sure a female patient is not pregnant and is using effective contraception.
• Start with a low dose and increase it slowly.
• Give a full trial of the medication (1–2 months).
• Attempt to taper and discontinue the prophylactic medication once headaches are well controlled.

The major drugs used for headache prophylaxis, recommended dosages, contraindications, and side effects are given in Table 18-2. Patients with frequent headaches may overuse analgesics or ergotamine. Overuse consists of using simple

▶ TABLE 18-2 Migraine Preventive Medications

Beta-Blockers

- Propranolol 40–320 mg/d. Effective. Side effects: drowsiness, night-mares, insomnia, depression, memory disturbances, decreased exercise tolerance.
- Atenolol 50–150 mg/d
- Nadolol 40–240 mg/d
- Timolol maleate 10–30 mg/d

Calcium Channel Blockers

- Verapamil 240–720 mg/d. Benefit may lag 3–4 weeks. Side effects: hypotension, edema, headache, constipation
- Nifedipine 30–180 mg/d
- Diltiazem 120–360 mg/d

Antidepressants

- Nortriptyline hydrochloride 10–125 mg/d. Effective independent of antidepressant effect
- Amitriptyline hydrochloride 10–300 mg/d
- Doxepin hydrochloride 10–150 mg/d
- Fluoxetine hydrocholride 20–80 mg/d. Fewer anticholinergic effects than tricyclics

MAO Inhibitors

- Phenelzine 30–90 mg. Side effects: hypotension, weight gain, edema. Requires close medical supervision and tyramine-free diet

Anticonvulsants

- Divalproex sodium (Depakote) 250–1500 mg. Side effects: GI distur-bances, sedation, tremor, hepatotoxicity, transient hair loss

Serotonin Antagonist

- Methylergonovine maleate 0.2–0.4 mg qid. Lacks significant peripheral vasoconstrictive effect
- Methysergide maleate 2–8 mg. Idiosyncratic fibrotic reaction (1/5000)

analgesics daily, combination analgesics containing barbiturates or sedatives more often than three times a week, or ergotamine tartrate more than twice a week. Overuse can produce chronic dependency headache with growing dependence on symptomatic medication and refractoriness to prophylactic medications. Stopping the overused medication frequently results in headache improvement following a period of increased headache ("analgesic washout period").

Referral

Referral should be considered if first-line therapies are ineffective, or the patient has a migraine syndrome unresponsive to usual medications. Individuals with headaches more frequent than once every couple of months probably require a neurological evaluation. Any patient with the "worst headache of their life syndrome" should probably be evaluated by a neurologist after diagnostic testing is obtained.

► REFERENCES

1. Headache Classification Committee of the International Headache Society. Classification and diagnostic criteria for headache disorders, cranial neuralgia, and facial pain. *Cephalalgia* 1988;8(suppl 7):1–96.
2. Andrasik F. Psychologic and behavioral aspects of chronic headache. *Neurol Clin* 1990;8:961–76.
3. Solback P, Sargent J, Coyne L. Menstrual migraine headache: results of a controlled, experimental outcome study of non-drug treatments. *Headache* 1984;24:75–8.
4. Silberstein SD. Office management of benign headache: the science and the art. *Postgrad Med* 1993;93:223–40.

OTOLARYNGOLOGY AND PULMONARY DISORDERS

Respiratory problems are found among all age groups. Chapter 19 deals with infections of the upper respiratory tracts, which are the most common reason for physician visits. Most are uncomplicated viral syndromes and are self-limited. Care of these individuals usually requires a physical examination to rule out more serious bacterial infections. The most difficult aspect of care is convincing patients unnecessary antibiotics that may cause more problems than viral syndromes. A brief review of diagnosis and therapy is presented.

Chapter 20 is in many ways a continuation of Chapter 19. The concept of sinopulmonary syndromes helps pull the respiratory system together and show how they complement one another. The diagnosis and treatment of pneumonia have changed to include the variable of host immunocompetence in treatment schemes. Additionally, characteristics of the organisms have changed, such as the newly emergent penicillin-resistant *Streptococcus* (possibly secondary to indiscriminate use of antibiotics for viral infections!). Asthma, or reversible bronchospastic disease, is reported to affect up to 5% of the population. Deaths from asthma have increased over the past 20 years. Recently, the use of over-the-counter medications for the treatment of bronchospastic episodes has been questioned. The philosophy of treatment is undergoing reevaluation. Anti-inflammatory medications such as steroids (inhaled and systemic) may replace bronchodilators in the future.

CHAPTER 19

Upper Respiratory Infections

The most common reasons for a patient to miss work or school and seek medical advice are the common cold and upper airway diseases. Most of these problems are caused by viral and bacterial infections. These infections are ubiquitous and are frequent in child care and close working environments. Most are spread by coughing, sneezing, and just talking. The most important aspect in caring for patients with upper respiratory infections is to resist the temptation to overtreat viral infections with antibiotics and to recognize the secondary bacterial infections that require therapy. Secondary bacterial sinusitis may occur in 0.5% of cases, and otitis media may occur in 2% of otherwise uncomplicated colds.

► COMMON COLD

The common cold may be caused by any of five or more different viral groups (the rhinogroup has more than 100 different antigenic types!), which limits the potential of developing a single vaccine. Despite progress in identifying organisms that cause "colds," many infections continue to defy identification.

Seasonal variation is important because most infections occur in the early fall to spring.

Diagnosis

Fortunately, in most cases, the patient is correct in self-diagnosis based on the upper airway symptoms of runny nose, scratchy sore throat, and mild fever (usually less than 100.4°F). Physical examination is helpful in distinguishing individuals who need more extensive testing for other diseases. A patient with a severely infected pharnyx with exudate should undergo evaluation for Group A β-hemolytic streptococcal infection. The ears should be observed for fluid, indicating serious otitis media, or erythema and inflammation, indicating acute otitis media.

Treatment

Many individuals suffering from a self-limiting viral infection can be treated easily with over-the-counter products designed to relieve symptoms. The use of nasal sprays containing phenylephrine and ephedrine should be limited to 4 days to prevent rebound hyperemia. Decongestants may help dry the upper airways and analgesics (aspirin, acetaminophen, and nonsteroidal anti-inflammatory drugs [NSAIDs]) are helpful in controlling fever and myalgia. Cough suppressants such as dextromethorphan and codeine are probably the most useful. Data on the effectiveness of vitamin C supplementation are unconvincing, but it causes no harm and many patients remain convinced of the benefit.

Referral

Patients with chronic sinusitis or with recurrent bacterial infections may require further evaluation to detect possible anatomical problems or immunological incompetency. These symptoms include continual pain in the location of the affected sinus and purulent bloody discharge. In most cases, the recurrence rate shortens between infections due to the nidus, which is never adequately drained.

▶ PHARYNGITIS

Pharyngitis may have multiple causes. Most often the cause is viral infection accompanying the common cold, but pharngitis also may be caused by aerobic and anerobic agents, including gonorrhea. In most cases, the important differentiation is to determine if Group A β-hemolytic streptococcus (*Streptococcus pyogenes*) is present and to prevent the occurrence of acute rheumatic fever and glomerulonephritis. Additional causes of pharyngitis that are important to identify are mononucleosis, human immunodeficiency virus (HIV), and herpes virus infections. A plan for the management of pharyngitis is outlined in Figure 19-1.

Diagnosis

Pharyngitis associated with common viral infections is classically described as a scratchy throat without severe pain and odynophagia. Fever, which occurs in acute bacterial infections, is not a prominent symptom with viral infections (except adenovirus infection). With viral infections, erythema may be

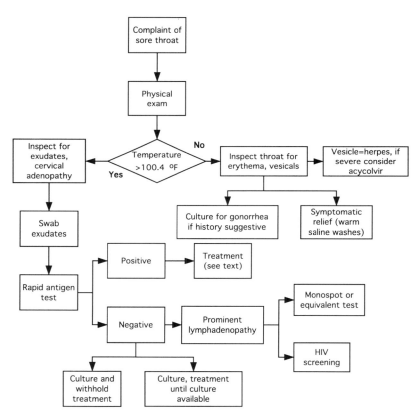

FIGURE 19-1. Algorithm for management of a "sore throat."

noted in the posterior pharynx, but a purulent discharge usually is not present. Anterior cervical adenopathy usually is present with bacterial infections and mononucleosis and not with viral infections. Herpes virus infections are associated with 1–2 mm vesicles and patchy ulcerations. Severe herpes virus infections may be accompanied by necrosis and a foul smell, typical of anaerobic infection. Unfortunately, pharyngitis found in HIV infections is nonspecific but may soon be followed by a maculopapular rash and lymphadenopathy.

Symptoms of streptococcal infections of the pharnyx are exudates, tender adenopathy (especially in the anterior cervical lymph nodes), and severe sore throat. Many patients have fevers exceeding 100.4°F. Unfortunately, some individuals become chronic carriers of streptococcus, and even though the results of identification techniques are positive, they may not have clinically significant disease.

Streptococcal diseases are usually diagnosed by one of two methods: rapid antigen detection tests or culture. Rapid antigen tests may be performed in a few minutes and have a specificity of over 90% (few false-negative results) but, depending on the method, a sensitivity of 60–95% (true-positive results). Traditional culture methods have a sensitivity of 90–95%, depending on technique, but require 48 hours for results to be available.

During physical examination, it is important to determine if the tonsils or pharynx is deviated and requires surgical drainage. If the decision is made to proceed with treatment, penicillin is the treatment of choice. Pen V-K, 250 mg four times daily for 10 days, remains the primary treatment, but benzathine penicillin, 1.2 million units, may be administered. First-generation cephalosporins may also be used but offer no advantage over the penicillins. Individuals who are allergic to penicillin may be given erythromycin, 250 mg four times daily, as an alternative.

Treatment should be initiated within 7 days of diagnosis to prevent the complication of acute rheumatic fever. Despite the decline in the incidence of acute rheumatic fever and the possibility of overtreating carriers of streptococcal infection, most clinicians would still recommend therapy, even in doubtful cases. In cases of primary gonorrhea with associated pharyngeal findings of erythema, culture and therapy are appropriate. With recurrent gonorrhea, culture of the throat along with cultures of the urethra, rectum, and cervix should be performed.

Referral

Individuals with deviated tonsils or with an abscess is the posterior pharynx should be referred to an otolaryngologist for urgent therapy. Many such infections will resolve with antibiotics but some will require surgery. Recurrent streptococcal infections should be referred to an allergist or immunologist to explore the possibility of other underlying etiologies causing recurring infections. Finally, streptococcus may be part of the normal flora in some individuals. In the absence of acute infection (e.g., swollen tonsils, pustulae, and fever) these patients should be observed.

▶ SINUSITIS

A common problem encountered in office practice is the patient with self-diagnosed "sinus problems," which may mimic multiple medical problems including headaches, dental pain, postnasal drainage, halitosis, and dyspepsia.[1] Sinus conditions may be secondary to primary problems anywhere in the upper respiratory system, leading to the concept of the sinobronchial syndrome.[2] The entire respiratory system (or sinobronchial region) may be infected by a particular virus or pathogen, but the most noticeable symptoms usually will be produced in one anatomical area. Therefore, when patients complain that an infection has "settled into" a region, they are correct!

Diagnosis

Most sinusitis is caused by a viral infection and is self-limited; however, secondary bacterial infections may result from the altered clearing mechanisms of ciliary function in the sinus cavity. The mucosa of the respiratory system may become inflamed by multiple infectious and environmental agents, such as atmospheric pollutants (especially tobacco smoke).[3] Other contributing factors include dental disease and anatomical deformities (septal defects). Most infections begin with a viral agent in the nose or nasopharynx, which blocks the ostia. The viral infection inflammation, which results in ciliary dysfunction in the sinus and a predisposition to secondary infection with bacteria. Clinical criteria for diagnosis include a purulent nasal discharge or cough lasting for more than 7 days,[4] maxillary toothache, poor response to nasal decongestants, change in color of nasal discharge, purulent discharge on physical examination, abnormal sinus transillumination, and abnormal sinus radiographs.[5]

The most common bacterial agents infecting sinuses are *Streptococcus pneumoniae, Streptococcus pyogenes, Haemophilus influenzae, Staphylococcus aureus,* and streptococci species. Opportunistic anaerobic bacterial infections are uncommon and usually associated with chronic sinusitis; however, in many acute cases mixed infections with both aerobic and anaerobic organisms are identified. Acute infection can occur in any of the sinuses but the maxillary sinus is most often affected because of the ease of obstruction of the small ostia in the nose. Fever, malaise, a vague headache, and pain in the maxillary teeth are usual early symptoms as well as a "full" feeling in the face with sudden motion. On physical examination, fever is absent in one-half of patients, and pain is exhibited by percussion over the malar area of the involved sinus. A purulent exudate from the nose may be present because of obstruction of the ostia in the nasopharynx.

Unless sinusitis becomes recurrent, imaging studies are not indicated. Plain films will reveal thickened mucosa early in the clinical course followed by opacification by inflammatory fluid. The final stages of infection usually demonstrate classic air–fluid levels on supine, upright, and lateral views. Cultures are rarely required and must be obtained by direct needle drainage to prevent contamination.

Treatment

Broad antibiotic coverage is effective in treating infections caused by most common aerobic and anaerobic agents and in shortening the course of disease. Ampicillin–clavulanic acid combinations, trimethoprim–sulfamethoxazole, and cephalosporins have proved effective. Decongestant drops such as phenylephrine are useful in shrinking the obstructive ostia but use should be limited to no more than 4 days. Therapies that may be helpful in relieving symptoms include facial hot packs and analgesics. Improvement should be apparent with 48 hours, but complete resolution may take up to 10 days with therapy continued for 14 days. In the absence of rapid improvement, another antibiotic preparation should be used based on presumed resistance. Treatment of sinus infections is important in controlling the spread of infection. Orbital cellulitis may lead to orbital abscesses, subperiosteal abscess in facial bones, cavernous sinus thrombosis, and meningitis by direct extension.

Chronic sinusitis usually results from repeated infections with inadequate drainage. Repeated attacks of acute sinusitis with incomplete resolution injure the surface ciliated epithelium, resulting in impaired mucus removal. A vicious cycle occurs starting with incomplete treatment, followed by reinfection and emergence of opportunistic organisms. Allergies may contribute to chronic sinusitis, with edematous mucosa and hypersecretion causing ductal obstruction and infection. Chronic cough and laryngitis with intermittent acute infections may also occur. Treatment involves controlling allergies and aggressive management of infections. Computed tomography (CT) scanning is indicated for evaluation for surgery. Endoscopic procedures have increased the success rates of sinus surgery.

Referral

Patients suspected of having chronic sinusitis should be referred to an otolaryngologist for evaluation and possible surgery. Cases that do not respond promptly to antibiotics may be complicated by osteomyelitis and obstructed ostia, leading to abscess formation. Surgical drainage and treatment with parenteral antibiotics may be indicated. Any cases that are suggestive of brain and dural abscesses require advanced imaging (CT or MR) and referral.

► BRONCHITIS

Acute bronchitis is an inflammatory condition of the tracheobronchial tree, occurring most commonly in winter from viral infections. The most prevalent viruses are the common cold viruses and *Mycoplasma pneumoniae*.

Diagnosis

Usually a cold or flu-like syndrome precedes bronchial symptoms by 3–4 days. Cough and sputum production may last up to 3 weeks in one-half of individuals and in one-quarter for 4 weeks.[6] Cough, hoarseness, fever, and sputum production are common symptoms. The prolonged nature of these infections results in patients demanding antibiotics to "clear up the infection." Sputum production may be prolonged in cigarette smokers and, because of chronic changes in the airway, they may have serious bacterial infections.

Physical examination should be directed at eliminating the presence of lower respiratory diseases, most commonly pneumonia. Isolated bronchitis is associated with diffuse upper airway sounds, usually coarse rhonchi and rales, without consolidation and alveolar involvement. Auscultation of the chest should carefully be performed to detect signs of pneumonia (fine rales, decreased breath sounds, and euphonia also known as E-A changes). Chest radiographs should be obtained if the diagnosis is unclear. As bronchitis resolves, sputum production may become more copious. Cultures of sputum are worthless because of contamination by the nasopharnygeal flora and the polymicrobial nature of infections.

Chronic bronchitis is a separate disease entity that usually is secondary to cigarette use. A strict definition is the presence of a productive cough from excessive secretions for at least 3 months of the year for 2 consecutive years. Chronic obstructive pulmonary disease (COPD), "blue bloaters," is one form of chronic bronchitis. Less common causes include chronic infections and inflammation from the inhalation of environmental pathogens. Incessant coughing with expectoration of sputum, usually after arising in the morning, is the cardinal manifestation of the disease.

Treatment

Treatment is directed at relief of symptoms such as control of fever with colds and flu and cough suppression. If the cause is thought to be mycoplasma, erythromycin is indicated. Antibiotic treatment should be reserved for defined infections such as pneumonia. The efficacy of expectorants has not been proved.

Referral

Patients who have had a cough for more than 1 month should be referred to a pulmonologist for a more extensive work-up, which may include bronchoscopy. Patients who have chronic bronchitis will usually have some degree of pulmonary compromise and require close follow-up. These patients may benefit from antibiotic therapy but require close monitoring. Because of the frequent exacerbations of bronchitis and the constellation of medications and hospital care required for many of these patients, a pulmonary physician is probably the best referral source.

▶ OTITIS SYNDROMES

Infectious otitis syndromes (otitis externa and otitis media) are fortunately less common in adults than in children. Certain conditions, however, may lead to ear-related problems.

Diagnosis

Otitis externa has multiple clinical syndromes and two are common in the obstetric and gynecologic age groups.

Acute localized otitis externa is associated with infection in a hair follicle in the external ear canal. This usually results in pustular formation with Group A *Streptococcus* and *Staphylococcus aureus* and may be associated with prominent cervical lymphadenopathy.

Acute diffuse otitis externa or swimmer's ear occurs in warm weather. An edematous, painful canal is noted on physical examination. The causative organism in most cases is *Pseudomonas aeruginosa*. Interestingly, this syndrome has been noted in persons using redwood hot tub systems.

Otitis media is an inflammation of the middle ear that is found most commonly in children less than 3 years of age. Occasionally, it is found in adults and is associated with viral syndromes such as the common cold. Signs of infection are severe ear pain and drainage, fever, and hearing loss. Infrequently, symptoms of vertigo and tinnitus are present. On physical examination, erythema and fluid below the tympanic membrane are present. Fluid may be demonstrated by the use of a pneumatic otoscope, which allows the introduction of air. By observing the absence of tympanic membrane motion, the presence of fluid is established. Fluid may remain for several months, however, even after successful treatment and is not a sole criterion of infection.

Treatment

If otitis externa arises from a pustula or furuncle, it is treated with local heat and antibiotics. Because *Staphylococcus aureus* is a causative agent, beta-lactam-resistant antibiotics (oxacillin or a first-generation cephalosporin) should be prescribed. Surgical drainage may be necessary if medical therapy is unsuccessful. In cases of acute, diffuse otitis externa, cleansing with 3% normal saline to rid debris, followed by a combination of rubbing alcohol and acetic acid (white vinegar), will usually be curative. Other possible treatments include ear drops formulated with corticosteroids and antibiotics that have been acidified.

Bacterial agents causing otitis media occur in the following order of frequency: *S. pneumoniae, H. influenzae,* and *Moraxella catarrhalis.* Recommended antibiotics are amoxicillin; for allergic patients (if no penicillin anaphylaxis history is obtained), the combination of erythromycin–sulfisoxazole or a cephalosporin may be substituted. In most cases, symptoms should resolve in 48 hours; if not, a beta-lactam-resistant organism may be responsible in those treated with amoxicillin. Amoxicillin–clavulanic acid combination or a first-generation cephalosporin should be substituted. The use of decongestants and antihistamines is usually recommended for relief of symptoms; however, there are no data to support that their use shortens the clinical course of disease.

Referral

In most cases, patients will experience relief of symptoms within days. Cases of acute localized otitis externa that do not respond quickly or appear to require surgical drainage should be considered for referral early in the course of the disease. Any patient who does not respond to treatment within 48 hours, or who does not respond to adjustment in the antibiotic agent used to treat otitis media, may require surgical drainage and should be referred to an otolaryngologist.

▶ REFERENCES

1. Evans FO, Sydnor JB, Moore WEC, et al. Sinusitis of maxillary antrum. *N Engl J Med* 1975;293:735–9.
2. Slavin RG. Sinopulmonary relationships. *Am J Otolaryngol* 1994;15:18–25.
3. Mabry RL. Allergic rhinosinusitis. In: Bailey BJ (ed). *Head and neck surgery—otolaryngology.* Philadelphia: Lippincott, 1993;290–301.
4. Shapiro GG, Rachelefsky GS. Introduction and definition of sinusitis. *J Allergy Clin Immunol* 1992;90:417–8.
5. Williams JW Jr, Simel DL, Roberts L, et al. Clinical evaluation for sinusitis. Making the diagnosis by history and physical examination. *Ann Intern Med* 1992;117:705–10.
6. Gwaltney JM Jr, Hendley JO, Simon G, Jordan WS Jr. Rhinovirus infections in an industrial population. II. Characteristics of illness and antibody response. *JAMA* 1967;202:494–500.

CHAPTER 20

Lung Disorders

Respiratory disorders are common causes of morbidity. Recently, it has been suggested that asthma is more common than previously recorded. Deaths from asthma have increased in the past 5 years and unsupervised use of over-the-counter medications have contributed to this increase. Pneumonia and therapy have also changed in the past 5 years with emerging resistance in some pathogens. The importance of host immunocompetence is currently recognized in antibiotic combinations.

► ASTHMA

Asthma is a clinical syndrome defined as recurrent airway obstruction that resolves either spontaneously or with bronchodilator therapy. The etiology remains unknown. Recently, asthma has been thought to be caused by an inflammatory response within the pulmonary tree rather than by a receptor imbalance as previously believed. Bronchoconstriction is the primary symptom of asthma and may be associated with hyperresponsiveness of the airways brought on by various physical and chemical stimuli or irritants.[1]

History

The male/female ratio is 2:1 in childhood, but the disorder is equally distributed between both sexes by age 30. Initial attacks usually occur before age 25 but may surface at any age. Attacks may be produced by a variety of stimuli including viral infections, air pollutants, respiratory allergens in susceptible individuals, blood transfusion reactions, food additives (particularly sulfites), exercise, occupational exposures, emotional stress, and medications (classically aspirin and beta-blockers in susceptible individuals).

Diagnosis

Dyspnea and wheezing are the clinical hallmarks of asthma. The symptoms may vary and range from a nagging chronic cough to life-threatening episodes of hypoxia from acute bronchospasm. Spirometry is useful when combined with provocative studies. The results are usually normal in asymptomatic patients, but the patient's condition may deteriorate quickly during an episode.

Pathophysiologically, an asthma "attack" consists of (1) various degrees of constriction of airway smooth muscle, (2) thickening of the airway epithelium secondary to airway smooth muscle contraction, and (3) accumulation of bioactive and inflammatory fluids in the airway lumen. Bioactive mediators and neurotransmitters such as histamine, acetylcholine, kinins, adenosine, and leukotrienes are important in mediating airway constriction. During acute airway obstruction (bronchospasm), airway resistance increases, which decreases gas flow rates in the bronchioles.[2] The decrease in air flow is more profound during the expiratory phase than it is in the inspiratory phase, resulting in air trapping and hyperinflation of the chest, which may be observed clinically. During the resolution phase of an attack, the large airways are the first to return to normal, followed by the peripheral airways.

The usual clinical presentation is progressive shortness of breath with associated symptoms of cough, wheezing, and anxiety. Vital signs usually reveal tachycardia with tachypnea. The rate of respiration varies from 25 to 40 breaths per minute. Associated physical findings are nasal flaring and chest wall hyperinflation diagnosed by increased resonance on percussion. Accessory neck muscle usage is common, and the affected individual is more comfortable sitting up rather than lying down. Respiration, wheezing, and rhonchi may be audible without a stethoscope. Auscultation will reveal musical wheezing, rales, and rhonchi in all lung fields. Paradoxically, decreasing wheezing may be the first sign of either impending respiratory arrest or resolution.

The results of pulmonary tests are abnormal, reflecting decreases in vital capacity, which is a measure of lung function, and ultimately respiration. Pulmonary function testing with spirometry is cumbersome and requires patient compliance, which is difficult to obtain during an acute attack. A more useful tool found in most emergency departments is a peak expiratory forced rate (PEFR) manometer (Figure 20-1). A piston-like device, pushed out of a calibrated tube, measures the force generated. These devices may be purchased by the patient and used to maintain a log of readings, which may be beneficial in difficult cases. During a usual bronchospastic attack, PEFR levels decrease. Once the attack begins to resolve, the PEFR level will increase and approach normal. Chest radiographs are rarely indicated unless there are symptoms suggestive of pneumonia. The role of routine assessment

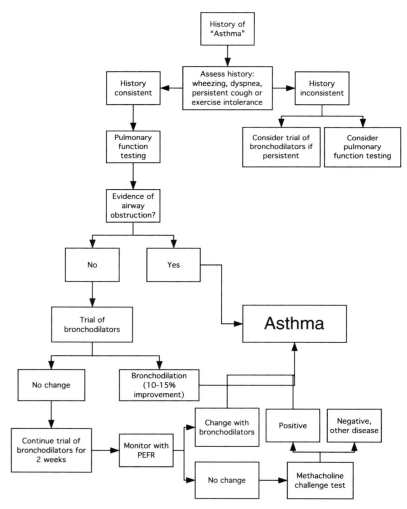

FIGURE 20-1. Algorithm for the management of asthma.

of arterial blood gases has been questioned, but this practice may be helpful in monitoring the severity of an attack. Pulse oximetry, which measures oxygen saturation in the blood (SaO_2), may be helpful in evaluating oxygenation and the clinical course; however, in densely pigmented individuals the measurements may be 2–5% lower than in those with light complexions.

Early stages of an asthma attack are manifested by a respiratory alkalosis. The $PaCO_2$ is usually between 25 and 35 mm Hg. The PaO_2 may range from 55 to 85 mm Hg on room air but is dependent on multiple factors. In most individuals an $SaO_2 > 90\%$ is adequate for normal metabolic function. As an attack worsens, the pH will "normalize" by a compensated metabolic acidosis (i.e., the $PaCO_2$ rises and is countered by a decrease in systemic bicarbonate). Therefore, a so-called normal $PaCO_2$ may signal exhaustion with impending pulmonary failure. "Status asthmaticus" is a clinical syndrome characterized by a sharp rise in $PaCO_2$ with a profound drop in pH brought on by the physical exhaustion of the patient. If a patient has other respiratory diseases, a history of prior intubation, or prolonged course over several days, tiring may require admission to an intensive care unit for closer observation.[3] Intubation and mechanical ventilation may be necessary with status asthmaticus.

Treatment

Bronchodilators are currently the mainstay of therapy in asthma, but anti-inflammatory agents may become more important in the future. Inhalation agents of the beta$_2$-agonists group are the most commonly prescribed.[4] The advantage of this group of medications is that they are topically applied and locally absorbed, which lessens systemic side effects. Stimulation of beta-2 receptors in the pulmonary tree results in dilation of constricted airways. Older inhalation agents such as epinephrine and isoproterenol stimulate both beta-1 and beta-2 receptors. Beta-1 stimulation results in uncomfortable tachycardia, which most patients find distressing. In the past decade beta-2 selective drugs were introduced; these drugs are better tolerated than beta-1 receptor stimulants and have an additional benefit of longer half-lives (approximately 5–6 hours compared with 2–3 hours). Preparations found in current clinical use are metaproterenol (Alupent® and Metaprel®) and albuterol (Proventil® and Ventolin®).

Inhaled beta$_2$-agonists are safer and better tolerated than subcutaneous epinephrine. A common problem with inhalation agents, however, is the proper administration of the agents. A certain degree of coordination is necessary to spray medication during inhalation. If improperly inhaled, the medication coats the posterior pharynx rather than bronchial tree. Patients should demonstrate proper inhaler usage. Individuals unable to coordinate the use of inhalers may require "spacers," which allow for better distribution of the medication.

Theophylline was the mainstay of chronic and acute therapy until the introduction of the beta$_2$-agonists. A significant problem with theophylline is a narrow therapeutic-to-toxicity range. Additionally, there is a wide variation in metabolism, which is influenced by factors such as age (younger patients metabolize the drug faster), concurrent medications (especially erythromycin and H$_2$-antagonists, which increase levels), and cigarette smoking (the clearance of drug is increased in smokers). Frequent monitoring of levels increases total cost, and toxicity is a constant concern. Despite these concerns, the condition of patients with nocturnal asthma may be better controlled with a single evening dose of a sustained-release preparation based on the theory that longer-acting agents "fill in" the gap between use of inhalation agents and allow for uninterrupted sleep.

A third group of medications are the anti-inflammatory agents that include cromolyn sodium (more correctly classified as a mast cell stabilizer), beclomethasone, and prednisone. Cromolyn sodium is useful *only* for maintenance and has no use during an acute episode. Beclomethasone is a topical steroid administered by inhalation that is useful for chronic therapy. The primary advantage of beclomethasone is that at most dosages it does not cause adrenal suppression. An annoying side effect of this drug is oropharyngeal candidiasis; with prolonged use, cataracts may occur. Candidiasis may be controlled with a spacer, which enhances medication delivery.

In severe or difficult-to-control cases of asthma, systemic corticosteroids may be utilized. Intravenous administration is usually necessary to control acute attacks and in emergency situations. Oral usage is necessary for long-term maintenance therapy. The mechanism of action is debated, but the primary action is based on decreasing inflammatory cell effects in the tracheobronchial tree. In acute situations, when patients fail to respond quickly to inhalation agents, corticosteroids should be administered intravenously. There is no consensus on dosage and schedules, but a dose of 20–80 mg of methylprednisolone is widely used, with 1 mg/kg repeated every 6 hours until the attack subsides. Once the patient responds, prednisone, 40–60 mg daily, is administered and the dosage is reduced by 5 mg daily until completed or the patient's previous baseline dose is reached.

Referral

The care of patients who have asthma that is chronically controlled by inhalation agents and who have occasional seasonal attacks is probably within the purview of the ob-gyn. Patients who have severe attacks more than once a year, require multiple medications and dosage schedules, are taking systemic steroids, or have multiple allergies should be treated by a pulmonologist. Additionally, individuals who have required care in an intensive care unit in the past will usually require greater expertise in management. In some individuals with chronic cough syndromes who do not respond to beta inhalation agents, referral for a more extensive work-up is warranted.

▶ PNEUMONIA

Pneumonia is an inflammation of the distal lung that includes the interstitium, terminal airways, and alveolar spaces. Multiple etiologies may be responsible for pneumonia including aspiration and infection with viral, protozoan, and bacterial agents. Aspiration pneumonia is usually the result of depression of the central nervous system, usually from drugs, alcohol, and anesthesia. Viral pneumonias are caused by a multitude of organisms such as herpes zoster, influenza A or B virus, parainfluenza virus, and respiratory syncytial virus. Most viral syndromes are spread by direct aerosolization of the environment from coughing, sneezing, and even talking. The incubation interval is only 2–3 days, followed abruptly by fever, chills, headache, fatigue, and myalgias. Despite the rarity of pneumonia in viral syndromes (1%), mortality rates may reach as high as 30%, especially in elderly and immunocompromised individuals. Secondary bacterial pneumonias are more common in the elderly.[5] The most lethal of pneumonias, regardless of age, is *Staphylococcus aureus* pneumonia, which may be preceded by a viral pneumonia. The best treatment for viral pneumonia is prevention by immunization. Patients who benefit most from immunization are those with chronic systemic diseases (primarily cardiac, pulmonary, and renal disease), diabetes mellitus, and connective tissue syndromes. In epidemics, amantadine has been used to treat nonvaccinated individuals.

History

For purposes of determining therapy and prognosis, bacterial pneumonias are classified as either community acquired or nosocomial. Recently, the American Lung Association has recommended four subgroupings of community-acquired pneumonia to better reflect demographic and disease trends.[6] These categories reflect patient age, immune status (especially related to human immunodeficiency virus infection), and the virulence of the organisms. Mortality from pneumonia still occurs and is more common in individuals suffering from chronic cardiopulmonary conditions, alcoholism, diabetes mellitus, malignancy, malnutrition, and renal failure. Poor outcomes are more common with two-lobe or more involvement, initial respiratory rate on presentation >30 breaths/minute, severe hypoxemia (<70 mm Hg), hypoalbuminemia, and septicemia.[7] Pneumonia is a common etiology in the development of adult respiratory distress syndrome (ARDS), which has mortality rates as high as 70%.

Diagnosis

Signs and symptoms of pneumonia vary, depending on the responsible organism and the status of the patient's immune system.[8] A strong index of suspicion is required in diagnosis, especially in elderly and immunocompromised individuals, who may have a more elusive presentation despite infection with common pathogens. In the elderly, especially since fever may be absent, the only clues may be sudden changes in mentation, confusion, or exacerbation of concurrent illnesses or chronic diseases. An increased respiratory rate of greater than 25 breaths/minute remains the most reliable sign of pneumonia. Mortality in high-risk groups is correlated most closely with the ability to mount normal host defenses such as fever, chills, and tachycardia.

Typically, pneumonia presents with high fever, rigors, productive cough, chills, or pleuritic chest pain. Chest x-rays are important in confirming the diagnosis and often show infiltration. In two-thirds of cases the most common organisms (in decreasing order) are *Streptococcus pneumoniae* ("pneumococcal pneumonia"), *Haemophilus influenzae, Klebsiella pneumoniae,* and Gram-negative and anaerobic bacteria.

Atypical pneumonias are insidious in onset, with moderate fever and lack of characteristic rigors and chills. Symptoms include a nonproductive cough, headache, myalgias, and mild leukocytosis. Chest x-ray shows a diffuse interstitial pattern rather than segmental involvement or bronchopneumonia. Affected individuals do not appear nearly as ill as the x-ray suggests. The most common etiologic agent is *Mycoplasma pneumoniae,* followed by the viral agents, then *Legionella pneumophelia* and *Chlamydia pneumoniae.*

Laboratory studies helpful in the diagnosis of community-acquired pneumonia are sputum Gram stain and, less frequently (and less accurately), sputum and blood cultures. The laboratory definition of an "adequate" sputum sample is more than 25 neutrophils and less than 10 epithelial cells per low-powered field on microscopic examination. Adequate sputum samples may be difficult to obtain, and most samples obtained by a patient using a sterile container results in spit, contaminated by oropharyngeal organisms. In most cases, an induced sputum sample obtained by respiratory therapists will have a higher yield.

Counterimmunoelectrophoresis (CIE) is an immunologic technique that uses the antigenic coating of a bacteria to produce an antibody-mediated response. It has been most useful in the identification of organisms in sputum, followed by those in urine and blood. The sensitivity and specificity of these tests vary according to the organism identified and the fluid or tissue used in diagnosis. Unusual organisms, such as *Legionella pneumophilia,* require direct fluorescent antibody staining of sputum or serological tests using sophisticated enzyme-linked immunoadsorbent assay (ELISA). *Mycoplasma pneumoniae* is suspected when diffuse bronchopneumonia is seen on chest x-ray and cold agglutinins are present with the appropriate clinical syndrome (i.e., headache, myalgias).

Diagnosis should focus on identification of the causative pathogen, to which therapy is then directed. *Streptococcus pneumoniae,* the most common community-acquired organism, has a classic presentation of sudden onset of fever, chills, and "rusty" appearing sputum with Gram-positive cocci ("coffee bean" cocci) on Gram stain. Bacteremia may be present in up to 25% of cases, and the diagnosis is occasionally established on the basis of blood cultures. The incidence of *Legionella pneumophilia* varies by region and is important to recognize because of the associated high mortality rate. The combination of high fever ($>40°C$), gastrointestinal and neurologic abnormalities, elevated liver enzyme levels and creatinine levels, and rapidly progressive abnormalities with multi-lobe involvement shown on x-rays should be helpful in the diagnosis.

Treatment

The mainstay of therapy is antibiotics. General measures in treatment are oxygen therapy and hydration. Pulse oximetry is useful if the patient is especially ill or has significant hypoxia (<70 mm Hg on arterial blood gas or SaO_2 <90 mm Hg). Criteria for hospitalization include respiratory distress, fever $>40°C$, metabolic abnormalities, especially metabolic acidosis, and altered mental status or meningeal signs. Chest physiotherapy is probably overprescribed and indicated only when overwhelming sputum production and ineffective cough are present.

In many cases, the exact identification of the organism cannot be determined, and empiric therapy should be initiated. Erythromycin is active against the three most likely organisms—*Streptococcus, Mycoplasma,* and *Legionella*—and should be used as a single agent for only immunocompetent and young patients. In elderly or immunocompromised patients, a second- or third-generation cephalosporin should be added for expanded Gram-negative coverage. Hospitalization is necessary for patients who are elderly, toxic, or immunocompromised.

Procaine penicillin G is no longer the drug of choice for pneumonia, even when treating streptococcal pneumonias. In most cases, a second-generation cephalosporin (cefuroxime axetil [Ceftin®]) 250 mg two times daily or amoxicillin–

clavulanic acid 500 mg three times daily without erythromycin is effective if a bacterial infection is strongly suspected. If the etiology is less certain and mycoplasma or chlamydial organisms are suspected, erythromycin, 500 mg four times daily, should be added to the regimen. The newer macrolides (clarithromycin/azithromycin) may be considered for monotherapy and may be an excellent choice in less well-defined infections. In cases where the patient has severe disease requiring hospitalization, parenteral second-or third-generation cephalosporins or ampicillin–clavulanic acid should be given in combination with erythromycin. Duration of therapy should be a minimum of 5 days (3 days afebrile) with uncomplicated pneumonia. Individuals who need to be hospitalized will require a minimum of 14 days of combined therapy, except with pneuminia caused by *Staphylococcus* and *Legionella* organisms, which require 21 days. Patients who are severely ill require extended combination regimens and should be referred.

Mycoplasma pneumoniae infections may be treated with erythromycin, 500 mg four times daily. Clinical severity will determine the rare need for hospitalization and intravenous antibiotics. *Legionella pneumophelia* usually presents with other systemic symptoms including severe headache and diarrhea. Erythromycin in high doses (2–4 g/day IV) is recommended. After the patient has been afebrile for 2 days, oral erythromycin, 500 mg four times daily, is begun for a total of 3 weeks. In severe, life-threatening infections, rifampin, 600 mg every 12 hours, is added to the regimen.

Finally, prevention of pneumonia with pneumococcal vaccines should be considered in high-risk patients such as the elderly (defined as >55 years of age), cigarette smokers, or patients with chronic pulmonary disorders. The vaccine is active against 23 different strains of pneumococci, which covers

85% of organisms cultured. The vaccine should be given prophylactically but can be given as a part of initial therapy. Repeat vaccination is suggested every 6 years because of potential poor antibody formation in the elderly. As noted above, these patients should be vaccinated with flu vaccine every fall prior to flu season.

Referral

Patients who do not respond to initial therapy may require more invasive techniques (transtracheal aspiration, thoracentesis, bronchoscopy, and lung biopsy) to determine a diagnosis as well as a change in antimicrobial agents. Elderly patients with multiple medical problems are difficult to treat because of their precarious physiologic balance. Treatment of immunocompromised patients (those with human immunodeficiency virus or who are dependent on steroids) in most cases requires extensive knowledge of extended microbiologic causes of pneumonia. Many of these patients require multiple combinations of antibiotics not frequently used in obstetrics and gynecology. Additionally, patients who are in septic shock, have signs of meningeal disease, or have compromised respiration will best be served by an internist or critical care specialist. Patients who do not respond in the first 48–72 hours may need hospitalization and referral.

► REFERENCES

1. US Department of Health and Human Services, National Heart, Lung, and Blood Institute. National asthma education program expert panel on the management of asthma. Guidelines for the diagnosis and management of asthma. 1991.

2. Burrows B. The natural history of asthma. *J Allergy Clin Immunol* 1987;80:373–7.

3. Nolan TE, Gallup DG. The gynecologist and surgical respiratory care. *Female Patient* 1992;17:15–28.

4. Barnes PJ. A new approach to the treatment of asthma. *N Engl J Med* 1989;321:1571–7.

5. Douglas RG Jr. Prophylaxis and treatment of influenza. *N Engl J Med* 1990;322(24):443–50.

6. American Thoracic Society. Guidelines for the initial management of adults with community-acquired pneumonia: diagnosis, assessment of severity, and initial antimicrobial therapy. *Am Rev Respir Dis* 1993;148:1418–26.

7. Woodhead MA, MacFarlane JT, McCraken JS, Rose DH, Finch RG. Prospective study of the aetiology and outcome of pneumonia in the community. *Lancet* 1987;1:671–4.

8. Farr BM, Kaiser DL, Harrison BD, Connolly CK. Prediction of microbial aetiology at admission to hospital for pneumonia from the presenting clinical features. *Thorax* 1989;44:1031–5.

INFECTIOUS DISEASE

Certain infectious diseases have either undergone a resurgence in prevalence or have traditionally been difficult to understand, especially because of confusion in interpretation of laboratory results. During the 1970s and early 1980s, the Centers for Disease Control and Prevention (CDC) were heralding the day in the first decade of the next century when certain infectious diseases such as tuberculosis would be eliminated.[1] Syphilis, even though present, had not been at epidemic proportions for over 20 years since the introduction of penicillin. Many of the scourges of humankind were at least under control. Then the human immunodeficiency virus (HIV) epidemic began. Many infectious diseases found an unwilling host—the HIV patient with the inability to adequately fight infection—despite adequate therapeutic agents.[2] Unfortunately, the inadequacies of underfunded public health departments and pharmaceutical research for development of newer agents have compounded the problem.

A review of hepatitis and the relationship and interpretation of infectious status by antigens and antibodies is included in Chapter 21. Despite the increased resurgence

267

of certain diseases, the incidence of other maladies is decreasing because of research into new vaccinations, most notably for hepatitis A and hepatitis B. As molecular biology provides new knowledge regarding the role of DNA and RNA in infectious disease, the potential for new vaccines rises. Research into HIV continues to move at a slower pace than wished, but new insight into viral replication and disease transmission is becoming available. In medicine, these areas of research may have the greatest yield.

Tuberculosis, the subject of Chapter 22, has also re-emerged as a significant pathogen. The recent epidemic is probably a combination of resistant organisms, immunocompromised hosts, and the growth of the homeless population. Interpretation of PPD skin tests has changed and reflects the changing demographics of tuberculosis and the role of immunocompromised hosts. Current guidelines stratify results of the skin test with the risk of the individual based on immunologic status and environmental risk.

Chapter 23 focuses on the diagnosis and management of syphilis. Questions on the identification and treatment of syphilis, once relegated to embarrassing students and residents on teaching rounds, are no longer such a rarity. Unfortunately, this disease has had a resurgence, and efforts should be directed toward preventing its spread through early detection and treatment.

Because information in these areas is extremely volatile, frequent updates by the practitioner are important.

The algorithms provided will hopefully help the reader logically approach these diseases and plan therapy, especially in the management of syphilis.

► REFERENCES

1. CDC. Update. Tuberculosis elimination—United States. *MMWR Morb Mortal Wkly Rep* 1990;39:153–6.
2. Selwyn PA, Hartel D, Lewis VA, et al. A prospective study of the risk of tuberculosis among intravenous drug users with human immunodeficiency virus infection. *N Engl J Med* 1989;320:545–50.

Hepatitis

$\mathbf{H}$epatitis is a common, highly infectious viral agent that is responsible for significant morbidity and mortality, especially in Asia and the Far East. The recognition of this potentially fatal disease, its diagnosis, and potential treatment have changed over the past decade. The ready availability of serum markers has made the diagnosis far easier, but the terminology for the various antigens and antibodies is confusing.

Viral hepatitis is a systemic infection that affects primarily the liver. Five types of hepatitis, which produce similar symptoms, have been described. A wide range of illnesses is present clinically, from asymptomatic to persistent infections, chronic liver disease, cirrhosis, hepatocellular carcinoma, and ultimately coma leading to death.

A major difficulty in interpreting results of hepatitis testing is the nomenclature. Each antigen and antibody are associated with infectivity or immunity and appear and disappear in a set sequence. The confusing number of serum markers produced by antigens and antibodies of the five recognized variants makes interpretation difficult. A key concept is that any marker for immunoglobulin (Ig) M is an acute marker, whereas IgG markers represent evidence of a more remote infection. The sequence, appearance, and significance of these markers in an emerging or chronic infection are important in counseling the patient with regard to infectiousness and potential treatments.

Antigenic/antibody testing is necessary to determine the infecting agent, establish a prognosis, and identify the need for immunization of close contacts. Constitutional signs of hepatitis include anorexia, nausea, vomiting, fatigue, malaise, arthralgias, myalgias, headaches, photophobia, pharyngitis, and occasionally croup. Symptoms precede jaundice by 1–2 weeks and typically diminish with jaundice. Physical findings of hepatosplenomegaly and cervical lymphadenopathy occur in only 10–20% of cases. The posticteric phase is variable and lasts anywhere from 2 to 12 weeks. Complete recovery occurs in 1–2 months in virtually all cases of HAV and HEV, whereas uncomplicated HBV and HCV resolve in 3–4 months.

Classically, an elevation in the SGOT and SGPT levels occurs, but their rise is variable during the prodrome of acute disease. Elevated bilirubin levels follow the initial rise in hepatic enzymes. Hepatic damage does not correlate with peak liver enzyme levels. These levels generally peak when the patient is icteric and progressively diminish during the recovery phase. Clinical jaundice becomes evident when the bilirubin level exceeds 2.5 mg/dL. The average rise in bilirubin is from 5 to 20 mg/dL. A simplified algorithm for the assessment of major hepatitis syndromes is found in Figure 21-1.

Care for acute hepatitis is primarily supportive. Hospitalization is not indicated unless there is evidence of dehydration, prolonged prothrombin time, or bilirubin levels greater than 15–20 mg/dL. Evidence of hepatic failure (encephalopathy) should prompt referral. Bedrest should be prescribed until symptoms abate; normalization of hepatic enzymes is not necessary. Alcohol should be avoided during the acute disease. Moderate alcohol use after recovery has not been associated with relapses or chronic hepatitis. Diet should not be modified.

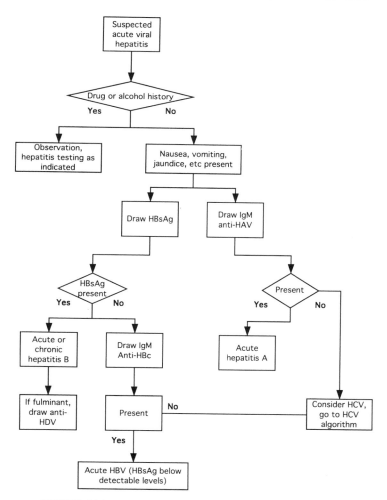

FIGURE 21-1. Algorithm for the diagnosis of hepatitis A and B.

Avoidance of some drugs is recommended, specifically chlor-promazine. Acetaminophen is preferable to aspirin to avoid gastric complaints. The use of oral contraceptives has not been proved deleterious to healing.[1]

► HEPATITIS A VIRUS

Hepatitis A virus (HAV) is an RNA virus occurring primarily in underdeveloped countries and transmitted via the fecal–oral route. The incubation period is approximately 15–45 days. Contaminated food, water, milk, and shellfish have been implicated in the transmission of HAV. The period of greatest infectivity is during the prodrome and early stages of the disease and rapidly diminishes once jaundice appears.

Diagnosis

The earliest serum marker is the anti-HAV IgM, which is indicative of acute infection. By 6 months this indicator of infection disappears and is replaced by the anti-HAV IgG. This marker will remain detectable indefinitely and accounts for resistance to reinfection. No carrier state for HAV infection has been identified.

Treatment

Because HAV is usually not transmitted by sexual contact, therapy is reserved for intimate contacts, such as household members and institutional patients. It should be initiated as soon as the infection is diagnosed. Hepatitis B immune globulin (HBIG) is used for prophylaxis against HAV and is given either prior to exposure or in the early incubation period (within 2 weeks after exposure). Prophylaxis is recommended for intimate contacts but not for casual exposures. It is administered in a dose of 0.02–0.06 mL/kg IM. The mortality rate for HAV is less than 0.1%.

A vaccine for HAV has been released for use in the United States. Candidates for vaccination may include those in military service abroad, those who travel to endemic areas, and health care workers. The recommended dose in adults is a single injection of 1440 ELIZA units (EL.U.), while in infants two injections of 720 EL.U. one month apart are recommended. Long-term antibody persistence is unknown at present.[2]

▶ HEPATITIS B VIRUS

HBV has been identified in most body fluids including saliva, tears, seminal fluid, cerebrospinal fluid, ascites, breast milk, synovial fluid, gastric juice, pleural fluid, and urine. It is usually transmitted by sexual contact, perinatal transfer, and percutaneous exposure to body fluids. The incidence of perinatal transmission is only 10% in the first and second trimester but rises to 65% in the third trimester.

Screening

Individuals at highest risk for HBV are health care workers, especially hemodialysis workers, Asians, Pacific Islanders, Alaskan Eskimos, Haitians, patients undergoing hemodialysis, household contacts of infected patients, individuals receiving multiple blood transfusions, pregnant women, and patients with multiple sexually transmitted diseases. In the event of acute disease, all close household contacts should be screened for evidence of immunity and should be vaccinated if necessary. Routine screening of pregnant women has been performed since 1988.[3] Individuals at risk should undergo screening on a routine basis if they have not been vaccinated or do not have evidence of immunity. Since 1993 routine universal vaccination at birth has been recommended. Vaccination may also be offered to adolescents with multiple sexual partners.

Diagnosis

The outer surface of the viron is identified by a surface-specific antigen designated HBsAg. The central core consists of DNA material and is identified as HBcAg. HBeAg is a serum marker associated with an intact viral particle and is a prognosticator of high infectivity. A 75–90% risk of perinatal transmission exists when the HBeAg is positive; however, when HBeAg is negative, the risk of transmission is less than 5%.[4] Antibodies to these antigens are termed anti-HBs, anti-HBc, and anti-HBe. Antigen formation is sequential: HBsAg forms first, followed by HBcAg, and lastly HBeAg. Replication of HBV occurs exclusively in the hepatocyte. The first antibody response is formation of an IgM anti-HBc, followed by anti-HBe, and finally anti-HBs. The immunity to HBV stems from anti-HBs, but the formation of anti-HBc is a reliable marker of resolving infection. Figure 21-2 shows a schematic illustration of infection and resolution. Patients failing to respond to antigen with the formation of appropriate antibodies become disease carriers.

Incubation of HBV occurs from 4 to 12 weeks. The HBsAg appears in the early acute phase and precedes the appearance of elevated liver enzymes. This serum marker re-

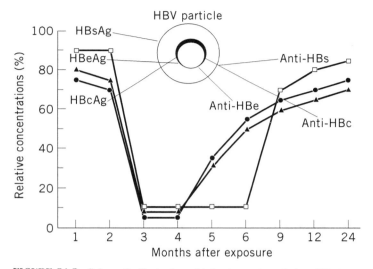

FIGURE 21-2. Schematic illustration of infection and resolution. HBsAg—hepatitis B surface antigen. First detectable response to HBV infection. HBcAg—hepatitis B core antigen. Sequestered in HBsAg coat and not routinely detected. The second response to HBV. HBeAg—hepatitis B "e" antigen. Third antigenic response to HBV. In protracted HBV infections, this antigen remains detectable. Anti-HBc—IgM antibody to HBc. First antibody response to HBV. Anti-HBe—antibody response to HBV. Indicative of low, but continued infectivity. Anti-HBs—antibody to HBs. Last antibody to appear and confirms immunity. (*Source:* Magann EF, Nolan TE. Hepatitis in the Ob/Gyn setting. *Female Patient* 1992;17:58–64. Used with permission.)

mains detectable through the icteric or symptomatic phase. After 1–2 months, HBsAg becomes undetectable and rarely persists past 6 months. If HBsAg persists beyond 6 months, chronic HBV infection or a carrier state may be present. Anti-HBc antibody is readily demonstrated in serum 1–2 weeks after the appearance of HBsAg. Detectable levels of the anti-

HBc antibody may evolve prior to other antibodies by weeks to months, making it the earliest marker to measure. Anti-HBc IgM is the predominant immunoglobulin in the first 6 months of the infection, followed by anti-HBc IgG, the predominating antibody after 6 months. The HBeAg appears shortly after HBsAg. In self-limited HBV infections, HBeAg becomes undetectable shortly after the peak elevations in aminotransferase activity. In protracted HBV infections, HBeAg may remain detectable.

Treatment

Because there is no specific therapy for hepatitis, the emphasis is on immunoprophylaxis. Prevention of further transmission should be discussed, especially the connection between blood and body secretions.

There are two acceptable approaches to prophylaxis for HBV infections depending on exposure history. Preexposure prophylaxis is useful in individuals at high risk of developing an infection, primarily the sexual partner. Three intramuscular injections of hepatitis B vaccine are given at 0, 1, and 6 months; pregnancy is not a contraindication to treatment. Postexposure prophylaxis consists of HBIG in a dose of 0.06 mL/kg given at the time of diagnosis and repeated 1 month later. In addition, hepatitis B vaccine should be given at 0, 1, and 6 months.

Newborn infants of HBsAg-positive mothers are given 0.15 mg of HBIG immediately after birth in addition to the routine series of hepatitis B vaccine started within 1 week of life. Currently, boosters are not recommended except in immunocompromised patients.

Referral

If hepatic enzymes return to normal levels with the usual progression of hepatitis markers, observation only is required. Ninety percent of patients with HBV recover without sequela except when infection is complicated by coexistent chronic hepatitis, advanced age, anemia, diabetes, congestive heart failure, or immunocompromise. The mortality rate for HBV is less than 1%. If evidence of carrier state exists (prolonged elevation of liver function tests, failure to convert antibody status), referral to a gastroenterologist is necessary for liver biopsy. Chronic carriers of HBsAg are at increased risk for hepatocellular cancer (hepatoma). There is no accurate laboratory test that allows accurate prediction of liver damage. Individuals who appear toxic and have mentation problems and acutely progressive courses may have fulminate hepatitis and should be referred. With coma, mortality is approximately 80%, and the only treatment may be liver transplantation.

▶ HEPATITIS C VIRUS

The virus responsible for hepatitis C virus (HCV) infection (formally classified as non-A, non-B or NANB) was first identified in 1988 with the discovery of an RNA virus. Two types have been described: the common blood-borne agent, which is closely associated with blood transfusion, and a water-borne variety associated with epidemics in India, Asia, and Central America. In the United States, 60% of HCV transmission is transfusion related, whereas the etiology for the remaining 40% remains unknown.

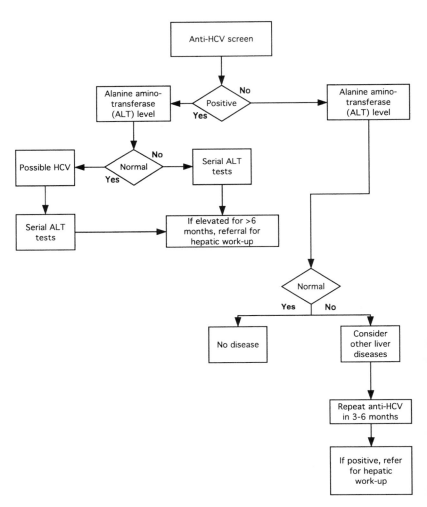

FIGURE 21-3. Algorithm for the diagnosis of hepatitis C.

Diagnosis

Testing methodologies to identify the virus are emerging but continue to be hampered by false-positive and false-negative results. The current diagnostic criteria recommended by the U.S. Food and Drug Administration (FDA) for interpreting laboratory tests for HCV are shown in Figure 21-3.[5] In the future, if the ELISA test for HCV is positive, a second test, the recombinant immunoblot assay (RIBA), may be performed. If the RIBA (currently not FDA approved) is positive, the chance of the individual having HCV increases greatly. Currently, there is no vaccination available. Despite a lack of data on transmission of the infection, shared usage of toothbrushes or razors by household contacts is discouraged, and safe sex with latex condoms is encouraged.

Treatment

Similar to HBV, prevention of blood and body fluid contamination from an infected individual is important to prevent transmission. Because the responsible virus changes rapidly, vaccine development is unlikely. Interferon therapy has been used in protocols for treating HCV and HBV infection. Although 50% of patients have some response during therapy, 50–75% relapse after therapy is terminated.

► HEPATITIS D VIRUS

Hepatitis D (delta hepatitis or HDV) is a defective RNA virus that requires HBV for replication and expression. The delta core is encapsulated by an outer coat of HBsAg. The virus can infect a person only by simultaneous infection with HBV or superinfection with preexisting HBV. Hepatitis D virus is transmitted predominantly by nonpercutaneous spread, usually by personal contact, Distribution of the delta strain is worldwide, with the virus being endemic in northern Africa, southern Europe, and the Middle East. The coexistence of acute HBV and HDV in a chronically debilitated patient carries a mortality rate of 5–20%. Fortunately, the occurrence of HDV is rare in the United States. If HDV is suspected, referral should be initiated because of the poor outcomes in this group of patients.

▶ HEPATITIS E VIRUS

Hepatitis E is thought to be a modified form, or endemic type, of hepatitis A. It is a self-limited disease transmitted by the fecal–oral route and has not been reported in the United States.

▶ REFERENCES

1. Schweitzer IL, Weiner JM, McPeak CM, et al. Oral contraceptives in acute viral hepatitis. *JAMA* 1975;233:979–80.

2. Clemens R, Safary A, Hepburn A, Roche C, Stanbury WJ, André FE. Clinical experience with an inactivated hepatitis A vaccine. *J Infect Dis* 1995;171 (suppl 1)S44–9.

3. Immunization Practices Advisory Committee. Prevention of perinatal transmission of hepatitis B virus: prenatal screening of all pregnant women for hepatitis B surface antigen. *MMWR Morb Mortal Wkly Rep* 1988;37:341–6,351.

4. Pastorek JG. Hepatitis B. *Obstet Gynecol Clin North Am* 1989;16:645–57.

5. *FDA Medical Bulletin* 1994;24(2):4.

CHAPTER 22

Tuberculosis

As recently as 1990, the Centers for Disease Control and Prevention estimated that tuberculosis (TB) would be eliminated as an infectious disease by the year 2010.[1] Social problems, such as the crowding of the homeless in inadequate shelters and a lack of surveillance for medication compliance in infected individuals, have contributed to the recent outbreak of tuberculosis.[1] Additionally, patients with HIV infection have increased the reservoir of patients infected with tuberculosis.[2]

Mycobacterium tuberculosis is commonly transmitted by inhalation of airborne infectious droplets. Droplets are produced when an infected host coughs (an average of 3000 droplets),[3] sneezes, speaks, or sings. The risk of disease transmission is enhanced by several factors such as the duration of exposure and the size and density of the infectious droplets. Droplets 1–5 um in size are implicated in disease transmission because they remain airborne for long periods and can avoid usual host defenses in the upper airway (primarily the mucociliary blanket), eventually reaching the alveoli.

The risk of infection to the exposed individual is determined by (1) the proximity of the contact, (2) the infectiousness of the source person, and (3) host defenses. Infectivity is greatest when acid-fast bacilli are present in the sputum, whereas individuals who only have positive culture results are less infectious. In the United States, an estimated 27% of household contacts of patients who have positive culture results become infected.[4] Once the tuberculosis organism enters the host, the infection develops in the lungs and then spreads locally to the hilar lymph nodes, followed by bacillemia.

Tuberculosis is classified either as an *infection* or as a *disease*. Tuberculosis infection is present when the organism is confined to the lungs. The asymptomatic patient with a positive tuberculin skin test and no systemic signs (such as weight loss, fatigue, etc.) would be considered infectious. Tuberculosis disease occurs when the infection extends beyond the lower lung and clinical illness ensues. Factors that increase the probability of progression include male sex (male/female ratio is 2:1), extremes of age, and suppression of cell-mediated immunity (HIV infection). Ten percent of infected patients ultimately progress to the disease state: 5% within the first 2 years of the initial infection and 5% from a reactivation of disease more than 2 years after the primary infection. Extrapulmonary disease is common in the lymphatic system, pleural cavity, musculoskeletal system, and genitourinary system.[5] Miliary, or generalized, tuberculosis occurs in approximately 9–10% of all patients with extrapulmonary disease.

Screening

The most common screening technique for tuberculosis infection is intracutaneous injection of purified protein derivative (PPD). Five tuberculin units (or TU) of PPD are injected in the volar aspect of the forearm, using a 26- or 27-gauge needle (the Mantoux technique). The dermis and vascular areas should be avoided during injection to avoid "wash out" of substrate. Reading of the area should be performed no less than 48 hours and no longer than 72 hours after injection. The Tine and Sterneedle (Heaf) tuberculin tests are multiple puncture techniques used for screening large populations. These tests may be associated with false-positive and false-negative results and should not replace the PPD test for screening.

Previously, an area of skin induration (not erythema) of ≥10 mm was considered a "positive" tuberculin test. The impact of HIV on cellular immunity resulted in a new scheme for interpreting PPD results. Risk factors and the measured skin induration now influence if prophylaxis is given. Following are indications for skin testing and risk factors for tuberculosis:

- Any sign or symptom suggestive of TB
- Known or suspected exposure to TB, especially for close personal or household contact
- Any risk factors for TB such as diabetes, drug abuse, alcoholism, immunosuppression, or HIV infection
- Hospital employees, nursing home workers, or prison workers
- Socioeconomic factors (poor nutrition defined as weight 10% below ideal body weight, crowded housing, homelessness)
- Race: African-Americans, Hispanics, Native Americans, Asian–Pacific Islanders

Patients with HIV as well as those who have a close household contact who has active tuberculosis or radiographic evidence of inactive tuberculosis are at high risk and should receive prophylaxis therapy for induration of 5 mm or greater. In individuals who are immigrants from areas endemic for tuberculosis, who are homeless, or who reside in a nursing home or a correction facility, a 10-mm induration is considered to be positive. In low-risk individuals (no risk factors for disease), a PPD induration of 15 mm is considered to be positive.[6]

Individuals less than 35 years of age who have been tested within the prior 2 years are classified as converters if they have an increase in skin reaction by 10 mm. Patients who are over age 35 are classified as converters if they have an increase of 15 mm. At age 35 the number of complications and side effects from isoniazid prophylaxis becomes significant.

Diagnosis

Patients with a positive tuberculin skin test should receive a focused physical examination for evidence of lymphadenopathy and abnormal auscultation of the lungs. A chest x-ray should be obtained (abdominal shielded after 12 weeks of gestation)[7] and the apical lung fields closely examined. Computed tomography and magnetic resonance imaging may be of value in defining calcifications, nodules, cavities, and vascular details in the lung. If genitourinary disease is considered, endometrial biopsies should be performed during menses for best yield. First-morning urine should be collected if urinary disease is considered.[8] Accessible lymph nodes should be aspirated.

Clinical disease may be confirmed by a combination of criteria. Acid-fast bacilli found in sputum, body fluids, or tissue are highly suggestive of infection. Findings of any two of the following three criteria may also be applied: (1) symptoms compatible with tuberculosis, (2) abnormalities detected by chest x-ray or physical examination (such as a draining cervical sinus of the neck), or (3) a positive tuberculosis skin test. The definitive diagnosis of tuberculosis is met when *M. tuberculosis* complex is identified by culture. Unfortunately, culture may take up to 6 weeks, which limits the timeliness of diagnosis. Newer DNA probes and microbiological techniques may soon be available to assist in diagnosis and management.

Prior to collection of samples, the laboratory should be contacted for any special instructions for sample preparation. Additionally, mycobacterial identification and sensitivity require a certain level of proficiency and fewer laboratories are offering these services.

Treatment

Prior to initiation of antituberculin therapy, the possibility of conception should be considered. Pregnancy should be delayed for individuals receiving therapy. Therapy is either prophylactic for skin test converters or therapeutic for established disease. Patients who are converters, without systemic or radiographic evidence of disease, may require therapy depending on age and risk factors. Current CDC guidelines are listed in Table 22-1.

Because adverse hepatic effects of isoniazid (INH) increase in individuals over 35 years of age, low-risk patients should not be treated.[9] The usual dosage of INH is 300 mg per day for 6 months unless the patient has concurrent HIV infection or radiographic evidence of old disease. Pyridoxine, 50 mg per day, should be given to avoid potential neuropathy associated with INH. In high-risk groups, 12 months of prophylaxis is recommended.[10]

Rifampin and additional agents (ethambutol, streptomycin, pyrazinamide) are added if there is progression to tuberculosis disease. Rifampin enhances cytochrome P450 metabo-

▶ **TABLE 22-1   Guidelines for Treatment of Tuberculosis**

Risk Category	<35 Years Old	>35 Years Old
Known risk factor (see text)	Treat at all ages if PPD reaction is ≥10 mm or patient is in high-risk group (see text)	
No risk factor, high-incidence group	Treat if PPD is ≥10 mm	Do not treat
No risk factor, low-incidence group	Treat if PPD is ≥15 mm	Do not treat

Source: CDC. Screening for tuberculosis infection in high risk populations: recommendations of the advisory committee for elimination of tuberculosis. *MMWR Morb Mortal Wkly Rep* 1990:39(RR-8):1–12.

lism and decreases the effectiveness of oral contraceptives; use of an alternative contraceptive is recommended during therapy. Active disease should be treated with two drugs, preferably isoniazid (300 mg/day) and rifampin (600 gm/day), with ethambutol (15 mg/kg/day) added if drug resistance is suspected.

The rates of INH-associated hepatitis by age group is (1) <20 years old, rare; (2) ages 20–35, 0.3%; (3) ages 35–50, 1.2%; and (4) over age 50, 2.3%.[9] Elevation of transaminase levels up to five times normal may occur in 10–20% of patients and should not be a cause for discontinuing medication.[10]

Referral

Patients in high-risk groups should be referred to public health officials for surveillance and follow-up. Patients requiring prophylaxis may receive routine follow-up care in a clinic, but protocols for observation should be initiated. Local public health guidelines are adequate. Consultation and possibly referral may be required for patients who have evidence of disease or who are in high-risk groups and may need therapy with two or three medications. Any patient with systemic illness (weight loss, fever, etc.) should also be referred to an internist with a special interest in tuberculosis.

► REFERENCES

1. Addington WW. Patient compliance: the most serious remaining problem in the control of tuberculosis in the United States. *Chest* 1979;76:741–3.

2. Selwyn PA, Hartel D, Lewis VA, et al. A prospective study of the risk of tuberculosis among intravenous drug users with human immunodeficiency virus infection. *N Engl J Med* 1989;320:545–50.

3. Rouillon A, Perdrizet S, Parrot R. Transmission of tubercle bacilli, the effects of chemotherapy. *Tubercle* 1976;57:275–99.

4. Comstock GW. Epidemiology of tuberculosis. *Am Rev Respir Dis* 1982;125:8–15.

5. Farer LS, Lowell AM, Meador MP. Extrapulmonary tuberculosis in the United States. *Am J Epidemiol* 1979;109:205–17.

6. CDC. Screening for tuberculosis and tuberculous infection in high-risk populations: recommendations of the advisory committee for elimination of tuberculosis. *MMWR Morb Mortal Wkly Rep* 1990;39(RR-8):1–12.

7. Hamadeh MA, Glassroth J. Tuberculosis and pregnancy. *Chest* 1992; 101:1114–20.

8. American Thoracic Society. Diagnostic standards and classification of tuberculosis. *Am Rev Respir Dis* 1990;142:725–35.

9. Kopanoff DE, Snider DE Jr, Caras GJ. Isoniazid-related hepatitis. A U.S. Public Health Service cooperative surveillance study. *Am Rev Respir Dis* 1978;117:991–1001.

10. Des Prez RM, Heim CR. *Mycobacterium tuberculosis.* In: Mandell GL, Douglas RG Jr, Bennett JE (eds). *Principles and practice of infectious diseases,* 3rd ed. New York: Churchill Livingstone, 1990;1877–1906.

Syphilis

The incidence of syphilis has risen at an alarming rate over the past decade, principally for the same reasons as those contributing to an increase in tuberculosis. The spirochete *Treponema pallidum* is responsible for syphilis, which is characterized by infrequent but severe and varied exacerbations. Recently, marked increases in the incidence of syphilis in reproductive age women have led to great emphasis on routine screening for all pregnant women. Pregnancy outcome, such as preterm labor, fetal death, and neonatal acquisition, may be influenced by maternal infection with syphilis.[1]

Treponema pallidum, found only in humans, has a spiral shape with corkscrew movements. It is too narrow to be seen by routine light microscopy and cannot be cultured. The organism remains alive just a few hours outside the body but much longer in blood. Spirochetes may enter through intact mucous membranes or a break in the skin.

Syphilis may involve every organ and is classified as a systemic disease. It is routinely divided into early and late syphilis. Early syphilis may be primary, secondary, and early latent. Late syphilis consists of late latent and tertiary.

Primary Syphilis. Following exposure to the pathogen, incubation times range from 10 to 90 days and are inversely related to the quantity of inoculum. The primary lesion, or chancre, appears as a single, painless ulcer at the site of entry. Chancres are highly infectious and may be found on the external genitalia, vagina, cervix, and extragenital sites including the mouth and anus. A confusing picture may arise if the original chancre becomes secondarily infected. Nontender regional lymphadenopathy may occur, especially in the groin. This primary chancre disappears spontaneously in 2–6 weeks without treatment.

Secondary Syphilis. Hematogenous spread of the spirochete with systemic involvement characterizes the secondary stage of infection. Secondary syphilis typically develops 3–6 weeks after the appearance of the primary lesion and remains for 2–6 weeks. The classic presenting sign in 70–100% of all cases is a maculopapular skin rash involving the entire body, including the palms of the hands, soles of the feet, and mucous membranes. When lesions coalesce in the perineum, they are referred to as condylomata lata. The rash of secondary syphilis is highly infectious because it consists of actively shedding spirochetes. Other signs and symptoms include generalized lymphadenopathy, malaise, fever, weight loss, and the "mouth-eaten" appearance of the scalp, eyelashes, and eyebrows. The lesions of secondary syphilis are mostly related to the deposition of immune complexes and resolve spontaneously.

Latent Syphilis. Latent syphilis is characterized by an asymptomatic period. It is classified into either early latent syphilis (duration less than 1 year) and late latent syphilis (duration greater than 1 year). Infection cannot be passed by sexual contact during this stage.

Tertiary Syphilis. Tertiary syphilis occurs in one-third of all untreated patients. Involvement of the cardiovascular, musculoskeletal, or central nervous system may develop from 1 to 20 years after the initial latent period. Cardiovascular lesions are characterized by aortic aneurysms and aortic insufficiency, whereas tabes dorsalis, paresis, and optic atrophy represent central nervous system manifestations. Neurosyphilis may occur at any stage but is most commonly seen in late latent syphilis.

Diagnosis

The most reliable method for the diagnosis of syphilis is the identification of the spirochete on darkfield microscopy. A fresh sample must be obtained and quickly examined. *Treponema pallidum* may be isolated from a primary syphilitic chancre, from the secondary skin rash, or from a condyloma latum. The major obstacles are cost of the test and the expertise needed for interpretation. Therefore, other less costly methodologies have been developed. Serologic testing is relatively inexpensive and readily available. Unfortunately, during the primary stage, both the nonspecific antibody tests and the treponemal tests may be nonreactive. Eventually, 100% of infected patients become positive after 4 weeks. Therefore, sexual assault victims should undergo repeat serology testing 30–45 days after the event.

Nontreponemal antibody tests detect IgG and IgM antibodies to cardiolipin, which is present on the spirochete. Three types of test are currently available: veneral disease research laboratory (VDRL), rapid plasma reagin (RPR), and automated reagin test (ART). These tests are not reactive until after the disappearance of the primary lesion. Once the test is positive, quantitative numbers are given for the amount of dilutions or "dils." Secondary or early latent syphilis usually his titers of 1:16 or greater; however, titers begin to fall in the late latent and tertiary stage and may become nonreactive. After treatment, titers should fall fourfold *over* 3–6 months. Therefore, retesting within 4–6 weeks may lead to the erroneous assumption that the patient is not responding. In most cases, the titer may return to 1:1 or 1:2 dils and may never become negative. The drop in titer to lower levels requires up to 1 year after treatment of primary syphilis and 2 years with secondary syphilis.

False-positive results may occur acutely with febrile illness, immunizations, or other spirochetal infections. Chronic false-positive results are associated with autoimmune diseases, narcotic addiction (which may be as high as 1:64), or chronic infections.

Treponemal antibody tests are used to confirm nontreponemal antibody screening tests. These tests include the fluorescent treponemal antibody absorption (FTA-ABS) and the microhemagglutination assay for antibody to *T. pallidum*. These antibodies remain throughout life and should not be used to monitor treatment but rather to confirm past or present disease. Since nontreponemal antibody tests may become nonreactive in late latent or tertiary syphilis, these tests may supplement screening in these individuals.

Cerebrospinal fluid may be obtained for the diagnosis of syphilis. There has been debate over the indications for lumbar puncture. The following indications may be used as a guideline, but consultation with an infectious disease specialist or public health department may be warranted:

Indications for Cerebrospinal Fluid Examination to Diagnose Syphilis

- Cranial nerve palsy
- Auditory symptoms
- Uveitis, neuroretinitis or optic neuritis
- Serum titers > 1:16
- HIV infection
- Gumma or aortitis
- Nonpenicillin therapy planned
- Duration of disease > 1 year

Spinal fluid abnormalities characteristic of neurosyphilis include white blood cell count elevated to >5 cells/mm³ and elevated total protein (>45 mg/dL) with normal glucose concentration.

Treatment

The CDC recommend penicillin as the first line of therapy for neurosyphilis and syphilis of pregnancy because it is the only effective treatment.[2] Other alternatives for the nonpregnant penicillin-allergic patients are tetracycline and erythromycin. Alternative regimens are inadequate in pregnancy, making the use of penicillin imperative. Pregnant women thought to be allergic to penicillin should first have skin testing performed to document the allergy and then undergo desensitization if present. Desensitization is accomplished with administration of

▶ **TABLE 23-1 Treatment Regimens for Syphilis**[a]

Primary

Benzathine penicillin G 2.4 million U IM single dose. Confirmed penicillin allergy: tetracycline 500 mg PO four times daily or doxycycline 100 mg PO twice daily for 2 weeks.

Secondary

Early Latent

Benzathine penicillin G 2.4 million U IM single dose. Confirmed penicillin allergy: tetracycline 500 mg PO four times daily or doxycycline 200 mg PO twice daily for 2 weeks.

Erythromycin 500 mg four times daily for 15 days in an immunocompetent host.

Late Latent or Unknown Duration

Benzathine penicillin G 7.2 million U total, given as three doses of 2.4 million U IM weekly. CSF normal with confirmed penicillin allergy: tetracycline 500 mg PO four times daily or doxycycline 200 mg PO twice daily for 4 weeks.

Tertiary

Benzathine penicillin G 2.4 million U IM q week for three total doses.

Neurosyphilis

Aqueous crystalline penicillin G 2–4 million U IV q 4 hours 10–14 days.
OR
Procaine penicillin G 2.4 million U IM daily, plus probenecid 500 mg PO (qid—both for 10–14 days.

U = units.

[a]*In pregnancy, late latent with abnormal CSF, or neurosyphilis, penicillin only!! Desensitization in necessary with confirmed penicillin allergy.*

100 U oral penicillin (V-K elixir), with a doubling of this dose every 15 minutes until 1,296,700 U is reached. Penicillin is given by injection 30 minutes later at therapeutic doses. This desensitization schedule is only necessary for the first injection. If a second injection and third injection are required, a minidesensitization regimen with 400,000 units oral penicillin (V elixir) is followed 1 hour later by injection.[3] Treatment regimens are outlined in Table 23-1.

The Jarisch–Herxheimer reaction is an acute, transient reaction noted following antibiotic therapy that may occur in 50% of patients undergoing therapy for primary syphilis. It is characterized by fever, chills, myalgias, and headache and may be more severe in secondary syphilis. The reaction is greatest in the first 12 hours after therapy and usually resolves after 24 hours. Fluids and antipyretics (Tylenol) are usually adequate treatment for this reaction.

After treatment, serial nontreponemal antibody titers are recommended. The same serological test (either the VDRL or RPR) should be performed and followed since each test is different. In primary syphilis, nontreponemal antibody titers should decrease fourfold after 3–4 months; if not, treatment failure or reinfection should be suspected. By 1 year, titers should be normal or no greater than 1:2. If disease continues longer than 1 year, titers should decline fourfold by 6–8 months and may require up to 2 years to become nonreactive. An algorithm of treatment and follow-up is outlined in Figure 23-1.

Referral

Depending on the expertise of the physician and the ability to perform a lumbar puncture, most of these patients may easily be treated by the obstetrician–gynecologist. Patients who have

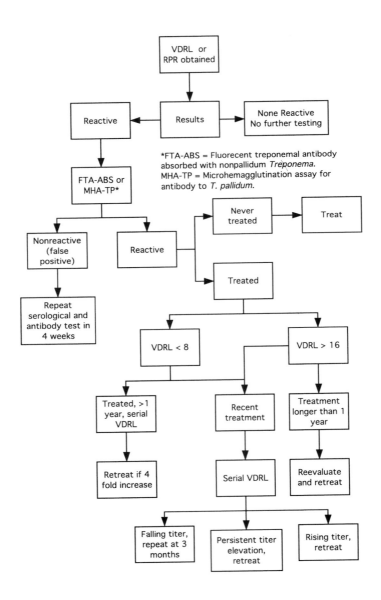

VDRL or RPR obtained

Reactive ← Results → None Reactive No further testing

FTA-ABS or MHA-TP*

*FTA-ABS = Fluorecent treponemal antibody absorbed with nonpallidum *Treponema.*
MHA-TP = Microhemagglutination assay for antibody to *T. pallidum.*

Nonreactive (false positive)

Reactive → Never treated → Treat

Treated

Repeat serological and antibody test in 4 weeks

VDRL < 8

VDRL > 16

Treated, >1 year, serial VDRL

Recent treatment

Treatment longer than 1 year

Retreat if 4 fold increase

Serial VDRL

Reevaluate and retreat

Falling titer, repeat at 3 months

Persistent titer elevation, retreat

Rising titer, retreat

questionable histories of penicillin allergy may be referred to an allergist to confirm the presence of an allergy. If desensitization is necessary, referral to an outpatient treatment area with easy access to inpatient services would be preferable.

▶ REFERENCES

1. Sexually transmitted diseases. In: Cunningham FG, MacDonald PC, Gant NF, Leveno KJ, Gilstrap LC III (eds). *Williams obstetrics,* 19th ed. Norwalk, CT: Appleton & Lange, 1993;1299–1302.

2. Centers for Disease Control. Sexually transmitted diseases treatment guidelines. *MMWR Morb Mortal Wkly Rep* 1993;42:27–46.

3. Wendel GD, Stark BJ, Jamison RB, Molina RD, Sullivan TJ. Penicillin allergy and desensitization in serious infections during pregnancy. *N Engl J Med* 1985;312:1229–1232.

GERIATRICS

The population of the United States is aging and increasing medical care will be rendered to geriatric patients. Chapter 24 is a review of the most common musculoskeletal disorders seen in a primary care practice. The impact of chronic diseases is just beginning to be appreciated. The ability to ambulate has important influence on the independence and long-term survival of many elderly patients. Chronic joint conditions, specifically osteoarthritis and rheumatoid arthritis, will have increasing significance. Joint replacement surgery has become widespread and increasingly sophisticated.

Chapter 25 is directed to urinary incontinence, a major problem in geriatric patients. The long-term use of an indwelling Foley catheter is probably responsible for more septic deaths than is generally appreciated. The number of women who will enter long-term care facilities will increase as the population bulge of the baby boomers occurs over the next three decades. The adult diaper industry barely existed 15 years ago but today has grown so dramatically that advertising dollars are spent in expensive media such as television. Much can be done for these patients, and it may be as simple as changing their living environment. The primary care physician will need to look at all aspects of a patient's medical care in order to assist them. These topics were chosen because of the number of patients they affect and the unique role of the gynecologist in relieving incontinence in the elderly.

CHAPTER 24

Musculoskeletal Disorders

Diseases of the joints and back are a cause of significant morbidity in women. Disorders of the back were once thought to be primarily a disease of men who were engaged in physical labor. As more women have entered the workplace, however, the prevalence of musculoskeletal (MS) disorders has increased. Many connective tissue diseases, such as rheumatoid arthritis (RA) and systemic lupus erythematosus (SLE), are more common in women than men. Additionally, the arthritides are chronic in nature and may last for decades. Osteoarthritis is a common affliction in women that may require surgery and joint replacement. Gout is fortunately uncommon in women, but it requires timely diagnosis to avoid more serious sequelae. Early recognition may help in decreasing morbidity from most connective tissue diseases. The gynecologist's role in the management of musculoskeletal disorders can be both diagnostic (SLE and RA) and therapeutic (osteoarthritis and back disorders).

▶ RHEUMATOID ARTHRITIS

Rheumatoid arthritis is the most common inflammatory disease of joints, affecting up to 1% of adults. Seventy percent of affected individuals are women, with peak incidence in the fourth to sixth decades of life. An important distinction to make is that RA affects the synovium early in the course of the disease and that early symptoms are related to inflammation around the joints, whereas joint and bone destruction are late manifestations of the disease. Although the exact cause of RA is unknown, the characteristic chronic inflammation of synovium is immunologically driven. An autoimmune phenomenon with tissue destruction is operative: T-cell immunity plays a central role in pathogenesis. In addition, RA is associated with particular inherited human leukocyte antigen (HLA-DR loci) alleles involved in the binding and presentation of antigen to T-lymphocytes.

Diagnosis

Rheumatoid arthritis should be considered in patients with polyarthritis in characteristic joints for 6 weeks or more. Pain and stiffness are accentuated in the morning or after prolonged inactivity (known as *gelling*). Stiffness in the morning or after gelling lasts for more than 30 minutes. Joints commonly involved in early RA are the proximal interphalangeal (PIP), metacarpal-phalangeal (MCP), wrist, knee, and metatarsal-phalangeal (MTP), but virtually any joint except those in the lumbar area may be affected. The involved joints may have visible erythema and are warm to the touch. Exerting any pressure over the afflicted joint will result in pain. Most patients with RA experience constitutional symptoms such as fatigue and malaise. In addition to the physical attributes of the joints, subcutaneous rheumatoid nodules may be found over pressure points such as the proximal ulna in 25% of patients.

The diagnosis of RA is based primarily on clinical findings.[1] Other supporting documentation may be confirmed by x-rays of the hand and joint showing characteristic joint space narrowing or juxta-articular erosions on the hand. Serology assessment to detect the presence of rheumatoid factor (RF) in serum is positive in 75% of patients in the first year of the disease. Early in the clinical course, however, the sensitivity of this test may be lower. Unfortunately, RF also is present in 15% of healthy elderly women, 35% of patients with SLE, and in patients who have other chronic inflammatory and rheumatic diseases.[2] Therefore, the diagnosis of RA should not be based on laboratory test alone but rather established in conjunction with associated clinical findings.

Psoriatic arthritis may be confused with RA, especially in younger patients with chronic polyarthritis. Usually, there is a history or presence of typical psoriatic skin or nail involvement (psoriatic nails are usually thin with severe pitting) in 90% of patients. Other differential points in the initial assessment include SLE, which may have symptoms of polyarthritis. Multisystem involvement is more common with SLE than with RA, and evidence of such involvement should be sought by a targeted history and physical examination. Although RA has long-term multiorgan sequela (aortitis, lung involvement), these findings usually occur after decades, not months. Laboratory testing for hematocytopenia and proteinuria as well as serology testing to detect factors specific to SLE may be helpful.

In older patients, osteoarthritis (OA) may be differentiated easily in most cases by its joint distribution (distal rather than proximal phalanges) and a lack of demonstrable inflammation. Arthritis may be caused by viral infections such as hepatitis B (more common in the elderly), parvovirus, and rubella. It is characterized by a symmetric joint distribution similar to RA but usually resolves within 2 months. Additionally, results of serology tests, such as those for hepatitis-associated antigens and antibodies, will be positive when arthritis is caused by infection.

Treatment

The goals of therapy are to reduce discomfort, maintain or restore function, and prevent joint destruction. Rheumatoid patients should perform daily exercises to maintain joint motion and muscle strength. Aerobic conditioning programs using low-impact regimens including walking, swimming, or stationary bicycling may help diminish discomfort. Assistive devices (devices that reach and grasp) may help make daily activities easier to accomplish and less stressful on inflamed joints. Orthotics may cushion the impact of subluxed metatarsal heads. Patients should be educated about the chronic and usually progressive nature of RA and its fluctuating course. Vocational and sexual counseling may be necessary in advanced cases.

Pharmacologic therapy is directed at decreasing inflammation in the joint. Therapy is usually initiated with a nonsteroidal anti-inflammatory drug (NSAID). There are different chemical structures of NSAIDs; if one medication is not effective, a different class should be tested. Approximately 20 NSAIDs are available in the United States with the exception of the nonacetylated salicylates.[3] The primary mechanism of action is to inhibit prostaglandin production, but NSAIDs also have antipyretic and analgesic activity. The choice of NSAID is usually dictated by cost, convenience, and side effects. The least expensive options include aspirin, ibuprofen, and indomethacin. Patients may prefer NSAIDs with longer dosing intervals for convenience and hence compliance. A therapeutic response should occur within a few weeks. Although no particular NSAID is consistently more effective than any other, different formulations have different half-lives and dosing schedules. Additionally, responses are idiosyncratic and thus vary greatly between individuals. Therefore, three or four sequential trials of different NSAIDs may be required. Approximately 30% of patients using NSAIDs will experience relief from pain and stiffness.

Nonspecific abdominal pain develops in 25–40% of patients while they are consuming NSAIDs. At the higher, chronic dosing required to treat RA, clinically significant gastric or duodenal ulcers develop in 2–4% of patients during the first year of therapy. Unfortunately, the correlation between abdominal symptoms and peptic ulcer is poor, and the first sign of problems may be an upper gastrointestinal hemorrhage or perforation of a hollow viscus. Risk factors for peptic ulcer disease should be documented and should include a history of peptic ulcer disease, older age, debility, glucocorticoid therapy, and higher doses of NSAID. Acute renal insufficiency is a side effect of NSAIDs that occurs as a result of inhibition of renal prostaglandins that regulate blood flow by vasodilatation or constriction. The resulting altered perfusion is generally mild and reversible. Patients at risk are the elderly or those who have preexisting renal insufficiency or decreased renal blood flow. For patients at risk, serum creatinine and potassium levels should be measured at baseline and repeated after 2–3 days (at approximately five half-lives or steady state). Hyperkalemia may develop in patients with sodium or volume depletion (dehydration), diabetes mellitus, or renal insufficiency, as well as in those receiving medications that raise serum potassium. Other adverse effects include bronchospasm in 10–20% of asthmatic patients and mild cognitive defects (in the elderly) or headaches in 5–10%.

After consultation with a rheumatologist, within months virtually all patients with RA will be treated with a disease-modifying antirheumatoid drug (DMARD) such as parenteral gold, methotrexate, sulfasalazine, or hydroxychloroquine in conjunction with a NSAID. In contrast to NSAIDs, which primarily treat symptoms, DMARDs may slow progression of RA. Disease-modifying antirheumatoid drugs have a slower response than NSAIDs. For example, 4–8 weeks of treatment with methotrexate are required to show benefit, and up to 6 months are required for injectable gold or hydroxychloroquine. Over one-half of treated patients derive benefit from any single agent, but, except with methotrexate and perhaps sulfasalazine, the effect wanes after several years. Glucocorticoids (e.g., prednisone, 7.5 mg or less per day) may be used as an adjunct while waiting for a response to a DMARD. Finally, intra-articular steroid use may be beneficial but should be limited.

Referral

Once arthritis is diagnosed and NSAIDs initiated, the patient should be referred to other health care providers. The DMARD agents have specific side effects that require close monitoring, and additional therapies (injections, orthopedic surgery) require subspecialty expertise outside the scope of a primary care practice. Optimal management is multidisciplinary and usually requires early consultation with physical therapy, occupational therapy, and rheumatology professionals. As disease progresses, orthopedic surgery is often needed to release contractures and increase mobility.

▶ **OSTEOARTHRITIS**

Osteoarthritis (OA), a degenerative joint disease, is the most prevalent form of arthritis. Prevalence of OA increases with age and body weight. At least 20% of the U.S. population have radiographic evidence of disease; fortunately, less than 250,000 are severely disabled. Osteoarthritis is characterized by erosion of cartilage at joint margins while the involved bone proliferates. The pathogenesis is multifactorial and involves biochemical, biomechanical, genetic, and immunologic factors.[4] Obesity is a major risk factor for OA of the knee, particularly in women.

Diagnosis

Patients with OA typically experience an insidious onset of pain and stiffness opposite to that of RA: it worsens after use and improves with rest. Morning stiffness may occur, but it lasts for less than 30 minutes. The most commonly involved joints include distal interphalanges, proximal interphalanges, basal joints of the thumb, cervical and lumbar spine, hips, knees, and the first metatarsal-phalangeal joints.

Physical examination may reveal painful joints with limited range of motion, firm bony enlargement or effusion in the joints, and bony crepitus. Typical signs of inflammation are minimal. Osteoarthritis may begin in a single joint but usually becomes polyarticular. Radiographic results correlate poorly with symptoms and clinical disease, demonstrating nonuniform joint space narrowing, subchondral bony sclerosis, and marginal osteophyte formation in the cervical spine. Generalized symmetric disease may be misdiagnosed as RA, particularly if serology results are false-positive. Clinical examination is probably more important than serology testing in connective tissue diseases.

Treatment

Osteoarthritis is a slowly progressive arthropathy that causes minimal disability when it is limited to small joints, usually in the hands. Despite the general overall favorable prognosis, knee or hip involvement may lead to total joint replacement in some cases. Treatment modalities in advanced cases include physical measures, adaptive devices, medications, and finally orthopedic surgery. Three to five times body weight is loaded across a joint surface when it is weight bearing. Patients with lower extremity OA may benefit from weight loss; if they are unable to lose weight, a cane, crutch, or walker may help stabilize the joint. Range of motion exercises may help to maintain flexibility and mobility. Heat or ice or both may provide relief of symptoms, especially when combined with exercise.

Pharmacologic therapy is indicated when discomfort becomes intolerable or interferes with daily life. Because there is little inflammatory component to acetaminophen in a dosage up to 4 g daily, it is preferred over NSAIDs. If acetaminophen does not control symptoms, a nonacetylated salicylate such as salsalate, 3–4 g daily, should be tried for approximately 1 month, followed by enteric use of coated aspirin, 650 mg three to four times daily. If pain control is not obtained with these medications, ibuprofen 1200 mg daily or other NSAIDs may be attempted. As discussed with RA, NSAID use in individuals with renal insufficiency and the elderly requires close monitoring for evidence of renal compromise.

Referral

Patients whose symptoms are not controlled with over-the-counter NSAIDs should be considered for referral. If advanced disease is present, referral to a rheumatologist to assess additional therapies or orthopedic referral for possible surgery is indicated. In advanced cases, joint prosthesis may allow normal function.

▶ GOUT

Gout is characterized by recurrent attacks of inflammatory arthritis precipitated by monosodium urate (MSU) crystals in synovial (joint) fluid. The cause of the joint inflammation is hyperuricemia, which leads to supersaturation of MSU within the joint and subsequent deposition in synovial tissue. When MSU crystals are injected into synovial fluid, they are phagocytosed by neutrophils that release lyosomal enzymes, causing inflammation. Hyperuricemia usually occurs secondary to decreased renal excretion of uric acid. Causes include chronic renal disease, lactic acidemia from alcohol ingestion, ketosis, dehydration, or drugs such as low-dose salicylate or diuretics. Many patients with gout have an idiopathic defect in uric acid excretion, and in 15% of cases gout is associated with idiopathic uric acid excretion, and in 15% of cases gout is associated with idiopathic uric acid overproduction. Gout is relatively rare in women, occurring in less than 1% in most series and usually in postmenopausal women. Uric acid levels increase during puberty in men, whereas in women this increase is usually delayed until menopause, leading to the age disparity in the onset of disease.

Diagnosis

Gout is divided into three clinical stages. Stage 1 begins with acute gouty arthritis, characterized by the rapid onset of severe inflammation of the fist metatarsal-phalangeal joint (big toe or thumb) and followed by inflammation of the ankle and knee in descending frequency of occurrence. Most attacks involve only one or two joints. Physical examination usually reveals marked, exquisite tenderness and florid inflammation and erythema, which may mimic soft tissue infection. Attacks may be precipitated by illness, surgery, trauma, or binge drinking. Untreated, attacks usually resolve within a few weeks and involved joints return to normal without permanent damage. The differential diagnosis includes infection and pseudogout. Synovial fluid analysis is necessary to distinguish these entities: gout has classic negatively birefringent, needle-shaped MSU crystals that may be undetected in 10–20% of cases. Serum uric acid plays no role in diagnosis and its presence may be misleading.

After the initial attack, most patients are asyumptomatic and the diagnosis may remain elusive; however, the majority of patients enter stage 2 and have a recurrence within 2 years. Unfortunately, as the disease progresses, the frequency, duration, and extent of attacks increase. If treatment is inadequate over a period of years, stage 3 results, which is manifested by tophaceous gout. Tophi, collections of MSU, develop over bony prominences such as the olecranon process, extensor proximal forearm, or other joints. Intra-articular tophi may insidiously erode subchondral bone and cartilage, resulting in permanent joint damage. Fortunately, with better recognition and therapy, such cases have become less common.

Treatment

Acute gout is often treated with NSAIDs, intravenous colchicine, and corticosteroids. Any agent is efficacious in up to 90% of cases. The earlier in the attack treatment is administered, the better it works. Used in anti-inflammatory doses, NSAIDs such as ibuprofen (800 mg three times daily) or naproxen (550 mg) work well unless they are contraindicated. Medication should be continued until the attack has completely resolved, up to 14 days. When given orally for acute attacks, high-dose colchicine produces gastrointestinal toxicity (usually profuse diarrhea) too frequently to be recommended. Intravenous colchicine has a relatively narrow therapeutic range; relatively small dosing errors may be fatal, limiting its usefulness. Corticosteroids may be given as prednisone, 20–30 mg daily, or intra-articularly to avoid systemic complications. Salicylate use should be avoided because the drug may alter the serum levels of uric acid and precipitate an acute attack. Alcohol use may precipitate attacks; use should be eliminated or closely monitored.

Once the acute attack has resolved, prophylaxis is indicated if recurrences occur frequently. Colchicine, 0.6 mg two times daily, is moderately effective in preventing recurrent attacks and produces minimal gastrointestinal toxicity. However, antihyperuricemic therapy has greater efficacy for long-term therapy. Individuals who underexcrete uric acid (defined as less than 600 mg of uric acid in a 24-hour urine collection) should be given probenecid (250 mg two times daily for 2 weeks, then 500 mg two times daily). In most cases, probenecid is benign, but it is contraindicated if renal insufficiency or a history of renal stones is present. Another effective medication is allopurinol, which is a xanthine oxidase inhibitor that decreases uric acid production. Allopurinol is also indicated in patients who overproduce uric acid or in those who have tophaceous gout. Regardless of the medication chosen, serum uric acid levels should fall below 6 mg/dL, which is the level at which intra-articular microtophi begin to dissolve. Colchicine (0.6 mg two times daily) must given concurrently during the first 6–12 months of antihyperuricemic therapy to prevent recurrent attacks.

▶ REFERENCES

1. Arnett FC, Edworthy SM, Bloch DA, et al. The American Rheumatism Association 1987 revised criteria for the classification of rheumatoid arthritis. *Arthritis Rheum* 1988;31:315–24.

2. Shmerling RH, Delbanco TL. The rheumatoid factor: an analysis of clinical utility. *Am J Med* 1991;91:528–34.

3. Brooks PM, Day RO. Nonsteroidal anti-inflammatory drugs: differences and similarities. *N Engl J Med* 1991;324:1716–25.

4. Liang MH, Fortin P. Management of osteoarthritis of the hip and knee. *N Eng J Med* 1991;325:125–7.

CHAPTER 25

Incontinence in the Elderly

The American population is aging, and management of conditions that are more prevalent among the elderly will account for an increasing proportion of gynecologic practice. Urinary incontinence is a common and underrecognized problem among the elderly. In 1988, the National Institutes of Health estimated that the cost of managing urinary incontinence approximated $10.3 billion per year. As the percentage of Americans over 65 years of age increases, the expense of managing incontinence will continue to rise. As many as one-third of women over 65 years of age suffer from incontinence and, among community-dwelling older persons, an estimated 15–30% have incontinence. Significant morbidity is associated with this problem because of skin changes resulting from chronic exposure to urine. In-dwelling catheters are convenient to use and make nursing care easier, but their use promoters sepsis. Physicians are reluctant to consider surgery in the elderly because of the misperception that the patient will not survive surgery. There is no evidence to indicate that these patients have an unusually high mortality rate from surgery for incontinence when they receive appropriate care.[1]

Changes that occur in elderly women make the lower urinary tract more vulnerable to dysfunction. Elderly women undergo changes that may alter the balance of urinary storage and emptying, resulting in the development of incontinence. The loss of estrogen in the menopause causes urogenital atrophy with thinning of the tissues in the bladder, urethra, vulva, and vagina. The trigone epithelium is also estrogen sensitive and becomes thin as estrogen levels decrease. With reduced collagen, connective tissue loses elasticity. Urethral support may be lost as connective tissue decreases and striated muscles atrophy. Genital prolapse worsens with age and may affect bladder sensation and bladder emptying. The neurologic effects of aging may lead to a reduction of adrenergic receptors and slowing of nerve conduction time. The combination of these factors results in decreased bladder capacity, increased sensitivity of the bladder and urethra, increased bladder neck mobility, and a decreased ability to suppress or initiate a detrusor contraction.

Changes in other organ systems also have effects on the lower urinary tract. Congestive heart failure and medications such as diuretics may increase urine flow. Elderly individuals produce proportionally more urine at night because kidney filtration decreases with age and rebounds at night, promoting nocturnal diuresis. Nocturia is exacerbated by postural redistribution of peripheral dependent edema. Neurologic compromise after stroke, Parkinson's disease, or dementia can contribute to a decreased awareness of bladder filling. Diabetes may increase urinary output by osmotic diuresis, and peripheral neuropathy may affect gait and thus the ability to reach the bathroom.

These conditions result in a decrease in bladder capacity and urethral closure pressure, lower urinary flow rates, and decreased detrusor contractile power in the elderly. Postvoid residual urine typically increases from 50 to 100 mL in the elderly; with decreased ability to suppress spontaneous detrusor contractions, incontinence may occur in previously continent women.

Stress incontinence is common in women over 65 and is estimated to be present in up to 45% of women depending on techniques used for diagnosis. Chronic pulmonary diseases are more prevalent in the elderly, which may exacerbate problems with stress incontinence. Detrusor instability and overactivity increase with age, which may reflect gradually increasing neuropathology. Patients with detrusor overactivity experience urge incontinence and may only partially empty their bladders. Elderly patients with incontinence from detrusor instability and hyperreflexia have little warning before urine loss occurs. Incontinence may present as sudden uncontrollable urine loss without prodromal urgency. Additionally, impaired mobility in the elderly exacerbates the problem.

Impaired detrusor contractility is a special problem in the elderly and has been labeled detrusor hyperactivity with impaired contractility (DHIC).[2] Although dementia, Parkinson's disease, and stroke contribute to DHIC, the condition is often seen without obvious neurologic compromise. Treatment is complicated because medications usually given for detrusor instability and hyperreflexia block detrusor contractility and may increase residual urine, hence worsening the condition. Periodic self-catheterization, combined with detrusor contraction-suppressing drugs, can be effective in managing incontinence but is often underutilized.

History

When discussing urinary complaints with elderly patients, the physician should attempt to resolve anxiety and reinforce how often these conditions occur.[3] Acknowledging the stress and embarrassment of urinary problems may resolve the reluctance to discuss these issues.

During history taking, important distinctions should be made between urge and stress incontinence.

The medical history is extremely important because medications may contribute to the development of incontinence. All medications used should be reviewed, including over-the-counter drugs. If possible, the patient should be encouraged to bring all medications for review.

Mental status is crucial to successful management; if the patient is unable to remember when she last voided or is unable to perceive dryness, treatment plans will be futile. Individual mobility and manual dexterity are important factors in evaluating the patient's ability to reach the bathroom and undress in a timely fashion. Undiagnosed or poorly controlled diabetes may be a cause of polyuria. Fecal incontinence is often associated with urinary incontinence and is a source of distress to the patient.

Diagnosis

The physical examination should target conditions such as congestive heart failure, arthritis, orthostatic hypotension, and peripheral edema, which contribute to continence problems. Special attention should be given to observing the patient for signs of stroke (lateralizing signs, gait disturbances, mobility and manual dexterity, and ability to perform higher mentation processes such as subtracting serial sevens). The patient may not realize a stroke has occurred or is purposely concealing it. The incidence of stroke increases with age, and a neurologic examination, including sensory and proprioception assessment, should be performed. The anal wink reflex may be absent in up to one-quarter of elderly women, but the bulbocavernosus reflex is usually intact.

The presence of a fecal impaction and occult blood in the stool should be investigated further. The patient should cough with a full bladder to demonstrate the presence of stress incontinence. Postvoid residual urine should be assessed at least once, and culture of the urine should be obtained to rule out an occult urinary infection.

The importance of fluid intake as it relates to urinary frequency cannot be overstated. The use of a frequency–volume bladder chart or diary should be instituted (Figure 25-1). The frequency–volume bladder chart provides information that may help target aspects of the work-up and therapy. Excessive fluid intake, inappropriate fluid restriction, the number of incontinent episodes, the patient's pattern of frequency and nocturia should be examined. A plastic collection "hat" that fits over the toilet bowl rim is useful in collecting and measuring urine volumes.

Urinary cytology should be assessed in patients with recent onset of frequency, urgency, and gross or microscopic hematuria to rule out urinary malignancy. Simple cystometry performed at the bedside may demonstrate unstable detrusor activity or stress incontinence in many cases. In the absence of classic symptoms of stress or urge incontinence, or if surgery is contemplated, more sophisticated urodynamic testing should be performed. Following are criteria for extensive urodynamic testing:

- Recent pelvic surgery
- Recurrent urinary tract infections

Name: _____

Date:				Date:			
Time	Intake	Output	Symptoms	Time	Intake	Output	Symptoms
Totals				Totals			

FIGURE 25-1. Frequency–volume bladder chart.

- Marked genital prolapse
- Stress incontinence (only if surgery is contemplated)
- Significant voiding symptoms
- Residual urine volume greater than 100 mL

Resnick[3] has devised the mnemonic DIAPERS to categorize the reversible causes of urinary incontinence commonly found among the elderly.

Delirium is disorientation that may be manifested by the inability to focus on sequenced tasks. These individuals may become incontinent because they do not perceive the need to void or perceive the need to maintain continence. Serial subtraction of sevens from 100 is an excellent test for delirium and higher cerebral function.

Infection can occur as a result of increased postvoid residual urine and changes in the bladder lining. Although symptoms of urinary tract infection are often present, many older women present with urinary incontinence and bacteriuria without dysuria.

Atrophic urethritis and vaginitis can lead to multiple disorders (senile vulvitis, loss of support of vaginal tissues) and trigger detrusor instability and loss of urethral coaptation, which may lower outlet resistance.

Pharmacological causes include many antidepressants and sedative-hypnotics, such as flurazepam (Dalmane), diazepam (Valium), and alcohol, which reduce patients' awareness of bladder sensation. Alcohol has a diruetic effect and is commonly used to induce sleep. Diuretics such as furosemide, ethacrynic acid, and bumetanide can produce incontinence by increasing urine output, which overwhelms the bladder. Antihistamines contained in over-the-counter cold remedies may change bladder and urethral tone. Narcotics and calcium channel blockers (nifedipine, diltiazem, and verapamil) may inhibit bladder contractility. Alpha-agonists (ephedrine, pseudoephedrine, phenylpropanolamine), found in cold remedies, increase outflow resistance and may cause acute urinary retention. Alpha$_2$-blockers (prazosin and terazosin) used in hypertension therapy will lower resistance in the bladder neck and urethra, precipitating urinary incontinence in some patients. Anticholinergic drugs may cause problems in patients with constipation or severe diverticulosis.

Psychological causes include depression and behavioral disturbances, which decrease patient motivation and may lead to decreased bladder awareness.

Excess fluid excretion can result from excessive fluid intake and various medical disorders, including venous stasis, congestive heart failure, and diabetes mellitus. Edematous states may also be caused by decreased albumin from malnutrition and use of nonsteroidal anti-inflammatory drugs and calcium channel blockers such as nifedipine.

Restricted mobility is a correctable cause of incontinence. Placing a portable commode within easy reach during the day may resolve the problem. Mobility can also be restricted by clothing, such as corsets and binders. Patients should be encouraged to wear comfortable, loose-fitting clothing that is easy to put on or remove and discouraged from wearing intertwined corsets, girdles, belts, garters, slips, and stockings.

Stool impaction can distend the rectum and pelvic floor, inhibiting parasympathetic innervation of the bladder and leading to urinary retention, voiding dysfunction, and incontinence. Proper diet, stool softeners, and disimpaction are useful.

Treatment

Treatment of contributing factors may improve continence significantly. Bowel problems should be treated by diet, stool softeners, and stimulants, as necessary. Diuretics should be used early in the day, and patients with peripheral edema should be instructed to restrict fluids and to elevate their legs in the evening. As stated earlier, clothing should be as simple as possible to allow quick and easy undressing (replace buttons with Velcro, etc.), and the placement of a commode in the living area during the day and at bedside at night may be helpful. Walkers and toilet seat adapters may promote mobility, and the installation of side-rails or side-bars to improve access will help in toilet use. The patient's inability to sit on the toilet with her feet on the ground has been shown to make voiding more difficult. Medication change to modify side effects from drugs is often useful. Diuretics or alpha-blockers such as prazosin, which are used for the treatment of hypertension, may be replaced by ACE inhibitors or other medications.

Genital prolapse often exacerbates incontinence and may be relieved with a pessary. Patients unwilling to use a pessary may facilitate bladder emptying by reducing their cystocele at the end of voiding. Estrogen replacement therapy should be administered when a pessary is used. It may also be initiated for other symptoms as needed. The effectiveness of estrogen use is best established in treating urge syndromes, and recent evidence confirms its usefulness in the treatment of stress incontinence.[4] Estrogen improves the thickness and vascularity of the vaginal epithelium and endopelvic fascia and improves tissue characteristics during surgery.

Medications useful for therapy include the alpha-agonists,

phenylpropanolamine (Ornade spansule) and pseudoephedrine (Dexatrim, Sudafed). Blood pressure should be monitored shortly after these medications are initiated because alpha-stimulants can increase blood pressure. Pelvic floor muscle exercise programs may be useful if the patient is well moti-vated and complaint. Postural changes to improve control or suppress urgency (including leg crossing, squeezing the thighs together, or bending over) should be discussed.

Criteria for deciding on incontinence surgery are the same as those for surgical treatment in younger women: Is the prob-lem surgically correctable? Do risks of surgery outweigh bene-fits? Are there overriding medical problems that preclude sur-gery? Can conservative measures be used to improve a patient's condition to the point where surgery is no longer desired? Consultation with a geriatrician or interested internist prior to surgery and in the immediate postoperative period will promote optimum patient care, particularly with regard to her medical status and fluid management. Because elderly women are predisposed to postoperative urinary retention, non-obstructing operations are preferred, and suprapubic catheters or clean intermittent self-catheterization should be used as ap-propriate.

Bladder retraining and behavioral modification are often as successful as drug therapy in elderly patients and avoid the potential side effects of medications. Patients selected for be-havioral modification techniques should be well motivated, able to learn, and willing to complete a training program.

Fluid management is key. Fluid intake should reach nor-mal levels (1500–2000 mL daily), especially in the presence of self-imposed severe restrictions. Many elderly patients restrict fluid intake to reduce urinary frequency; unfortunately, highly concentrated urine may be even more irritating to their bladders than a larger volume of more dilute urine. At least 1500 mL of fluid should be consumed daily, with consumption evenly distributed throughout the day except 3 hours before bedtime.

A specific timed voiding schedule, which may be augmented by an alarm, may be beneficial. A bladder chart should be maintained and checked periodically. A 2-hour voiding interval is probably a reasonable period.

Anticholinergic medications may be used in elderly patients after attempts have been made at bladder retraining and behavioral modification. Drug dosages should be reduced in elderly women because of impaired renal clearance and the possibility of producing urinary retention. Propantheline bromide (ProBanthine) may be administered orally in doses of 7.5–15 mg three times daily and increased to higher doses or four times daily administration. Oxybutynin chloride (Ditropan) should be given orally in doses of 2.5 mg two times daily with the dose increased slowly to three times daily or to 5 mg at similar intervals. Because Ditropan has a short half-life, it may be used episodically to help the patient remain dry for important events. Imipramine (Tofranil) is useful because it increases urethral tone, as a result of its alpha-adrenergic stimulating properties, and relaxes the detrusor, as a result of its anticholinergic characteristics and effects on the central nervous system. Low doses (10 mg orally three times daily) should be used and increased carefully because of potential orthostatic hypotension and cardiac arrhythmias.

Catheters, despite their ease of use for nursing personnel, may result in urosepsis, a major cause of morbidity in patients in nursing facilities. Absorbent pads and barrier creams can protect the skin and reduce the odor of urine without catheter use. Clean intermittent self-catheterization (or intermittent

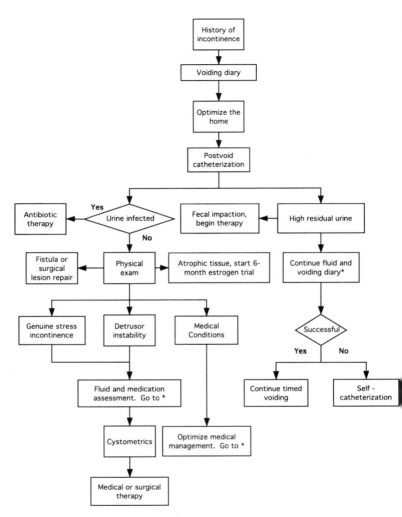

FIGURE 25-2. Algorithm for management of geriatric urogynecologic disorders.

catheterization by nursing personnel) may be useful.[5] This underutilized technique is often never considered; thus the patient is not given the opportunity to try it. Although infection rates with intermittent self-catheterization are higher in nursing homes than in the home setting, they still pose less risk of infection than chronic in-dwelling catheterization.

Referral

Home health care nursing may be helpful in implementing many of the strategies that involve behavior modification or patient motivation. Patients who may benefit from surgery may best be treated with the help of an internist, especially in evaluating medications for the variety of underlying problems that may exist in the elderly (Figure 25-2). In many cases, a urogynecologist may be helpful in evaluation of patients for surgery and performing the surgery. Referral for anorectal manometry to evaluate pelvic floor dysfunction and anal incontinence may be helpful in some situations.

▶ REFERENCES

1. Nolan TE. Surgery in the elderly: lowering risks by understanding special needs. *Postgrad Med* 1992;91(2):199–208.

2. Resnick N, Yalla S. Detrusor hyperactivity with impaired contractile function. An unrecognized but common cause of incontinence in elderly patients. *JAMA* 1987;257:3076–81.

3. Wall LL, Norton PA, DeLancey JOL. Special considerations in the elderly. In: Wall LL, Norton PA, DeLancey JOL (eds). *Practical urogynecology.* Baltimore: Williams & Wilkins, 1993; 316–31.

4. Fantl J, Wyman J, Anderson R, Matt D, Bump R. Postmenopausal urinary incontinence: comparison between non-estrogen-supplemented and estrogen-supplemented women. *Obstet Gynecol* 1988;71:823–8.

5. Whitelaw S, Hammonds JC, Tregellas R. Clean intermittent self catheterisation in the elderly. *Br J Urol* 1987;60:125–7.

▶ Index

Diuretics:
cholesterol and, 101
gout and, 311
hypertension treatment, 83–85
pregnancy and, 85
urinary incontinence and, 316,
321, 323
Divalproex sodium, 232
Diverticulitis, 62, 160
Documentation, change therapy, 39
Domestic violence, 18, 212
Doxazosin, 87
Doxepin, 219, 232
Ductography, 139
Duodenal ulcers, 307
Dymelor, 115
Dyschezia, 164
Dyslipidemias, 74
Dyspareunia, 217
Dysphagia, 180–181
Dysthymia, 215

Eating disorders, 24, 214, 216, 222
EDTA, cholesterol measurement, 98
Elavil, 219
Elderly (ages 65 and above):
calcium channel blockers and,
87–88
constipation in, 163, 166
death, leading causes of, 71
depression in, 212
diabetes screening and, 116
morbidity, leading causes of, 71
musculoskeletal disorders in,
309–314
pneumonia in, 260, 262
screening recommendations for,
68–71
thyroid disease in, 121
urinary incontinence, 316–327
Electrocardiograms, 33, 81
Electroconvulsive therapy, 217
Electroencephalogram (EEG), 216
ELISA (enzyme-linked

immunoadsorbent assay):
defined, 15
hepatitis C virus (HCV), 281
pneumonia, 261
Enalapril, 84
Encephalopathy, 272
Endep, 219
Endocrine disorders:
diabetes mellitus, 107–117
diagnosis, 27–28
thyroid disease, 119–129
Endocrinopathies, 109
Endogenous pathway, 94, 96
Endoscopic retrograde
cholangiopancreatography
(ERP), 175
Endoscopic sphincterotomy, 176
Endoscopy, 149, 181
Ephedrine, 322
Episodic tension-type headaches
(ETTHs), 223
Ergotamine, 229–230
Erythema, 195, 239–240
Erythromycin, 100, 195, 247, 256,
262–263, 296
Escherichia coli, 161–162
Estrogen, 120, 171, 316
Estrogen replacement therapy, 99,
196, 323
Ethacrynic acid, 321
Ethambutol, 287
Ethanol intake, 98
Ethinyl estradiol, 196
Ethnic minorities:
diabetes in, 108, 110
gallbladder disease, 171
lactose intolerance, 160
nutrition counseling and, 24
Euphonia, 246
Exercise:
cardiovascular fitness, 31–32, 74
cholesterol level and, 98
constipation and, 166–167
diabetes and, 113